INDIGESTION

INDIGESTION

*Living Better with
Upper Intestinal Problems
from Heartburn to Ulcers
and Gallstones*

Henry D. Janowitz, M.D.

OXFORD UNIVERSITY PRESS
New York   Oxford

Oxford University Press

Oxford   New York   Toronto
Delhi   Bombay   Calcutta   Madras   Karachi
Kuala Lumpur   Singapore   Hong Kong   Tokyo
Nairobi   Dar es Salaam   Cape Town
Melbourne   Auckland   Madrid

and associated companies in
Berlin   Ibadan

Copyright © 1992 by Henry D. Janowitz

First published in 1992 by Oxford University Press, Inc.,
198 Madison Avenue, New York, New York 10016-4314

First issued as an Oxford University Press paperback, 1994

Oxford is a registered trademark of Oxford University Press

Library of Congress Cataloging-in-Publication Data
Janowitz, Henry D.
Indigestion: living better with upper intestinal problems
from heartburn to ulcers and gallstones /
Henry D. Janowitz,
p.   cm.   Includes index.
ISBN 0-19-506308-2
ISBN 0-19-508554-X (PBK)
1. Indigestion—Popular works.   2. Stomach—Diseases—Popular works.
3. Peptic ulcer—Popular works.   I. Title.
[DNLM: 1. Digestive System Diseases—diagnosis—popular works.
2. Digestive System Diseases—therapy—popular works.
3. Dyspepsia—diagnosis—popular works.   4. Dyspepsia—therapy—popular works.
W1   145   J34i]   RC827.J36   1992   616.3/32-dc20
DNLM/DLC   for Library of Congress   92-19172

4 6 8 10 9 7 5

Printed in the United States of America

For my grandchildren,
Kita Rose and Andrew,
with the hope they will never
need this book

Preface

My previous book, *Your Gut Feelings,* dealt with problems of the lower intestinal tract—the pathway from the small intestine on down to the colon. It was designed to answer my patients' questions about preventing and taking care of such disorders as the irritable bowel syndrome, ulcerative colitis, Crohn's disease and diverticulitis, and such difficulties as diarrhea and constipation.

Its reception by the public, judging from their letters, and the interest of my patients, judging from their sharp questions, led me to recognize their needs and desires for similar information and guidance about the disorders of the equally important upper gastrointestinal tract—the pathway from the mouth to the upper small bowel.

If almost half of my patients complained about their bowels, an equal number consulted me because of a whole conglomeration of complaints which they lumped together as "indigestion." When one considers the complex interplay of forces which begins with the start of a meal and includes the swallowing function of the esophagus, the mechanical movements of food through the upper and lower bowel, and the part that the liver, gallbladder, and pancreas play in this digestive ensemble, it is no wonder things can go wrong from time to time and lead to indigestion, heartburn, and any number of other complaints.

Best known to the general public is *peptic ulcer,* which strikes about 10 percent of the general population at some time in their lives. Aside from the price of human suffering and the loss of days at work, the cost of medication presents a staggering sum. In fact, the most widely prescribed class of drugs throughout the world is the group of drugs that block the formation of stomach acid, the so-called histamine II blockers. The group now includes Tagamet®, Zantac®, Pepcid®, and Axid®. There is also a new type of acid-blocking agent, Prilosec®. But in saying farewell to indigestion, we are really addressing the problem of *dyspepsia,* the more technical term for dysfunctions of our digestion rising from the upper digestive tract.

This book offers advice on how to avoid and take care of this whole complex of disturbances we call indigestion. To set the stage, I begin with an overview of how this conveyor belt operates—from the mouth until the digested food reaches the small intestine where it is absorbed. I feel it is important for you to have some knowledge of this process in order to understand how your discomfort arises and what your physician needs to do to diagnose its causes correctly. Most people know more about what is under the hood of their cars than about what makes up their own innards!

We then turn to the basic problems of indigestion, trying to sort out the different vintages. It is more than a semantic exercise in defining terms; it is an attempt to pinpoint the search and zero in on the correct target. Because of the array of digestive symptoms and the interplay of several organs, a variety of standard tests are used by your physician in a diagnostic search to detect what may be wrong with the structure of your upper intestinal organs or, equally important, what may be wrong with their function. For this purpose, a whole host of new imaging techniques and inventions are at hand. I devote considerable space to these diagnostic devices because they are so valuable; you need to know their value and their risks, their advantages, as well as their drawbacks. Obviously, not only cost is important here; your informed consent to undergo these procedures is critical in the management of your discomfort. I try to answer the eternal question we all raise: How much testing must I have before my physician begins to treat me?

Turning to the core of this book, the ever-present problem of heartburn, secondary to inflammation of the esophagus (esophagitis), and its relation to the anatomical defect of a hiatal hernia, is obviously closely related to the problem of ulcers and touches on the serious problem of chest pain not resulting from heart disease. Distinguishing chest pain of cardiac origin from chest pain of a noncardiac condition is frequently difficult and crucial for proper diagnosis if we are to avoid making cardiac cripples out of individuals whose chest pain originates in the esophagus.

Continuing with the core of the book on specific problems, I consider *peptic ulcer* next by virtue of its frequency and complications. It deserves our attention, including a discussion of what we know of its causes, its prevention, and our best methods of treatment. As important as the healing of an ulcer, whether it resides in the stomach or duodenum, is the necessity of maintaining that healing. The recent rediscovery of the fascinating organism, *Helicobacter pylori,* formerly known as *Campylobactor pylorides,* is an intriguing chapter in the history of modern ulcer disease. This organism appears to play a role in ulcer formation and ulcer relapses.

The damaging and injurious effects of modern-day medications on the stomach is a subject of vital importance in an aging population, especially for those taking a good deal of aspirin and aspirinlike drugs (usually called nonsteroidal anti-inflammatory drugs, or NSAIDs), which include ibuprofen (Motrin®) and its relatives, in particular those used for the treatment of arthritis. With the risk of complications in the upper gut in the form of bleeding and perforation, it is necessary to bear in mind the medications you take and recognize that doses of these medicines can wreak havoc on the lower bowel too, especially in the case of ileitis or colitis.

When your symptoms sound like ulcer, yet our imaging techniques fail to reveal an ulcer, as is often the case, this condition of *non-ulcer dyspepsia* (as it is called) presents us with diagnostic and therapeutic puzzles; however, it is no less serious because we cannot give it a proper Latin name.

Indigestion has always been associated in the layperson's mind with *gallbladder disease.* Do we ignore the discovery of gallstones, try to discover them, dissolve them, or attempt to crush them by a shock wave from the outside? Do we remove them and the gallbladder through a formal abdominal surgical operation or, in the latest fashion, attempt to snatch the gallbladder and its stones through minor incisions in the abdominal wall by using a laparoscope and a TV monitor? The chapter devoted to the gallbladder offers some guidelines to help you make an informed decision in consultation with your doctor. I also address some fallacies associated with gallbladder disease.

Diseases of the liver could fill an entire volume, but in this book I focus on problems associated with the appearance of *jaundice*—the yellowing of the skin—which results from the blockage of the flow of bile from the liver or gallbladder. The bile is deposited in the skin and appears responsible for the attendant itching. Jaundice is discussed in connection with the gallbladder and *disorders of the pancreas.*

Disorders of the pancreas have an ominous sound, but *acute* and *chronic inflammation of the pancreas,* which is discussed in a separate chapter, prepares the reader for the chapter on *maldigestion, malabsorption, and malnutrition* of our diet, with their attendant disruption of the normal course of digestive events.

The core of the book on specific problems is rounded off by a review of three further problems: food allergy and food intolerance, the aging gut, and the brain-gut connection. Unfortunately, food intolerance and food allergy, which both play a role in causing digestive disorders, are still not completely understood and often invoked out of ignorance. In Chapter 12 I point out some of the misconceptions in this area and suggest how the reader can sort out what may or may not be a food allergy.

As members of an aging population, we are all interested in what the "tincture of time" does to our upper gastrointestinal tract. I summarize age-related changes in the various organs that may contribute to indigestion and recommend some guidelines for readers, middle-aged and older.

The role of emotions in disorders of the upper gastrointestinal tract—the brain-gut connection, as I call it—is a fascinating subject worthy of its own chapter.

Some mundane, although equally vexatious, symptoms and problems find their place in the Appendix. There belching, nausea and vomiting, dry mouth and bitter taste are discussed, along with difficulty in tasting, lump in the throat, swallowing difficulties, the strange effects of diabetes on the gastrointestinal tract, as well as the controversial "yeast connection."

If this book guides without being dictatorial, enlightens without overwhelming its readers with facts, informs without frightening, and encourages a cooperative dialogue between patient and doctor, then it will have accomplished its author's intent. I have not wanted to make part-time doctors out of its readers, but to encourage the development of an informed, medically literate public that modern medicine needs in this complex technological age.

New York   H. D. J.
January 1992

Acknowledgments

As always, this book owes most to my patients who asked me the hard questions; the "worried well" asked the sharpest ones.

Dr. Blair Lewis furnished me with the view of the endoscope. Dr. Daniel Maklansky provided me with the radiograph. And Dr. Jose Romeu gave me the film of the ERCP.

I owe Joan Bossert, my editor, a special debt of gratitude for her skillful editing and sharp pencil, which helped enormously.

Contents

III Appendix

Figures

Tables

I

INTRODUCTION

1

The Upper Digestive Tract

An Overview of How It Works and What It Does

You might suppose that enjoying and digesting a meal would be a relatively simple matter. Yet the process is a complicated one and begins with the thought, smell, and sight of food which sets in motion the intricate mechanics of the entire upper gastrointestinal tract.

In the mouth, chewing begins the process of grinding and chopping our food into sizes suitable for swallowing. This mechanical process, as well as the chemical composition of our diet, starts the salivary glands secreting their saliva. This fluid moistens the food, thus easing our swallowing, and allows the tastebuds of the tongue to sense the flavor of our diet. Very little of the chemical changes that make the diet suitable for absorption into the body take place in the mouth. Only *amylase*—a starch-splitting enzyme—is there, but has little time to act before the meal passes rapidly from the mouth through the esophagus and into the stomach (*Figure 1*).

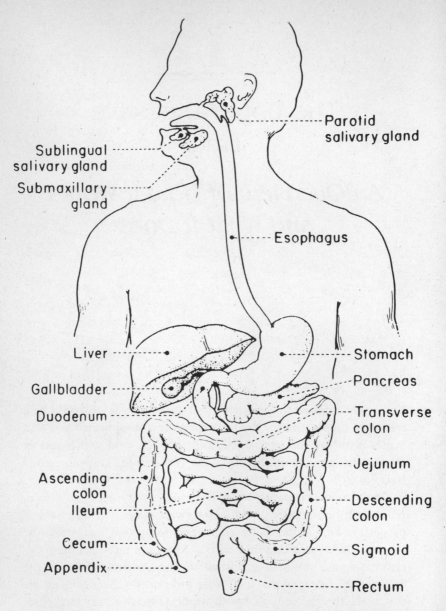

Sublingual salivary gland

Submaxillary gland

Parotid salivary gland

Esophagus

Liver

Stomach

Gallbladder

Pancreas

Duodenum

Transverse colon

Jejunum

Ascending colon

Ileum

Descending colon

Cecum

Sigmoid

Appendix

Rectum

FIGURE 1. Diagram of the gastrointestinal tract from the mouth to the rectum.

Swallowing and the Esophagus

Of course, for food to get into the esophagus we must swallow it. This is done by muscles, some of which are under our voluntary control and some of which contract or relax automatically. Swallowing starts when the liquids and the solids of our meal are pushed into the back of our throat—the pharynx—by the tongue. This part is voluntary and sets off an involuntary chain of events that transports the contents of the throat, through the esophagus, into the stomach. But little material moves in this chain by gravity—that is, by the weight of the food—only something heavier than water, such as the barium used in X-ray examinations, can move through its sheer weight. Things move through the esophagus because they are pushed by contractions of the esophageal muscles.

Imagine the entire intestine as an empty tube surrounded by coats of muscles. In successive waves, these muscles contract in a rhythmical fashion called *peristalsis*. While the esophagus is moving things along, it must also prevent material from backing up and re-entering the throat (regurgitation). And, at its lower end, it prevents the contents of the stomach, expecially its acid, from backing up into its own interior. So the esophagus has two "gatekeepers": one at the upper end—the upper esophageal sphincter, and one at the lower end—the lower esophageal sphincter. They see to it that the traffic generally moves in the right direction.

Although the esophagus usually deals with one-way traffic, remember it must be flexible enough in its function to allow for vomiting of an irritant up from the stomach. So the sphincters or "gates" can open and close appropriately, and usually remain closed until material needs to pass through. This happens by virtue of the natural resting contraction of their muscle fibers and the influence of their controlling nerves.

The *control* of this complex action is activated by the swallowing center of the brain. In the course of normal swallowing, neural messages are sent ahead, relaxing the lower esophageal sphincter even before the food arrives, so that the trap door is opened in advance. In addition to this mechanism, a number of substances in the diet and chemical messengers (hormones) released from the upper intestine can help to open or close the lower sphincter. All of this preparatory action—which I have simplified a great deal—takes place without our being aware of the process. Obviously things can go wrong in this complex chain and can lead to a variety of unpleasant sensations that will form the core of the discussion in the chapters that look at difficulties in swallowing and especially "heartburn."

How the Stomach Works

When our meals, partially prepared by chewing and moistening by saliva in the mouth, enter the stomach after a rapid passage through the esophagus, the work of digestion has only just begun as the enzyme amylase in our saliva begins to break down the starch of our diet into sugars.

The Mechanical Work of the Stomach

In the stomach the important work of grinding and mixing of food into a soft mush takes place so that the first portion of the upper small intestine—the duodenum (*Figure 2*)—can receive and handle the now comfortably sized and conveniently liquified meal. This breaking down of the larger particles of the diet is helped, not only by the liquids we swallow as we eat and drink and by saliva, but also by the large amount of dilute hydrochloric acid that the lining glands of the stomach add to this slurry, especially while we are consuming a tasty meal. In the presence of the acid, the lining of the stomach also secretes a group of digestive enzymes called *pepsins*, whose job is to break down the proteins of our diet (vegetables, meat, poultry, fish, etc.) into their constituent parts—the amino acids—which will be absorbed further down the digestive tract in the small intestine (see *Figure 1*).

The secretion of acid fluid and the digestive enzymes, the pepsins, is accomplished by specialized cells that are in the inner lining

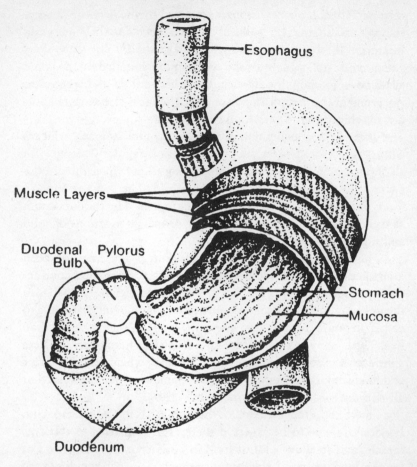

Figure 2. Details of the stomach and its muscles.

of the stomach (the mucosa). The mixing, grinding, holding, and emptying of our food from the stomach are accomplished by the thick wall of the stomach with its surrounding muscles, for the stomach is really a specialized muscle for pushing its contents along by muscular contractions. Unlike the contractions of the voluntary muscles of the arms and legs, for example, the contractions of the stomach are automatic and not under our conscious control. The regulation of these contractions is governed by the nerves and nerve cells within the stomach wall and impulses traveling through nerves that leave the brain and enter the spinal cord. At the same time, "stop" and "go" signals for the stomach are sounded by the upper intestine—especially the duodenum—which sends its messages to the stomach by neural impulses and chemical messengers (hormones) that travel in the blood to the stomach.

Fats in the duodenum slow the emptying of the stomach, which is why in some societies fatty food or cheese is regularly served with alcoholic beverages to slow down the speed at which the alcohol passes into the gut and thus into the blood. The concentration of foods and the salt content of our meals are sensed by the duodenum as well, whose job it is to see that the proper proportions of solid and liquid food move along.

When our stomach is empty and our body has not been nourished for some time, the stomach begins its rhythmical contractions, called "hunger contractions," which we may feel as pangs in the upper abdomen, signaling to the brain that the time has come to be fed. In our affluent society where we eat by the clock, rather than from need, many of us have never experienced a hunger pang. These contractions also account for stomach noises, which result when air and fluid are jostled around inside us—somewhat like the noise that air and fluid make in radiators.

A most important function of the stomach is its storage capacity. Food needs time to be digested there. The stomach can relax its muscles and so allow a lot of food to be eaten in a short period of time as food waits to be prepared for its further passage down the gut. It is easy to see how, if something goes wrong or interferes with this relaxation, we may experience unpleasant sensations. I discuss this in more detail in Chapter 6.

If you visualize the stomach, which is one organ, as working in two sections—*the upper portion,* the portion which receives the food first, called the *fundus,* and the *lower portion,* which leads into the duodenum and which mixes and grinds the food up, called the *antrum* or *antechamber*—it will help you visualize the well-integrated action of these two stomach sections. Their work goes on all the time, and when we get no unpleasant sensations from the stomach, we can assume that the process is proceeding normally (see *Figures 2* and *4*).

The *fundus* is responsible for holding and storing food and regulating the speed at which liquid exits the stomach; the solid portion of the food leaves in a different way and at a different speed. The *antrum* mixes and grinds the diet and then squirts small amounts in a thin stream into the duodenum—a beautifully orchestrated and programmed sequence in this conveyor belt. In addition to the secretion of water and hydrochloric acid by the stomach and its addition of pepsin to digest protein, the stomach lining cells also secrete the material called *intrinsic factor*—a complex material which attaches to the vitamin B12 in our diet, permitting it to be absorbed lower down in the ileum by another series of coordinated steps; B12 is crucial for the manufacture of hemoglobin (the red oxygen-carrying pigment of our red blood cells).

The Digestive Work of the Stomach

So far we have mainly been discussing the mechanical work the stomach does as it mixes, grinds, and moves the food along. Now we have to sketch briefly how the stomach pours out its liquid contribution which carries on the digestive work. the surface layer of the stomach—the mucosa—is lined with a single layer of defensive cells coated with a jellylike mucus that protects the stomach wall itself—a defensive platoon, so to speak, set against the offensive platoon of acid and pepsins, the digestive ferments. The surface lining cells pour out this coating of mucus, while the pepsin and acid are secreted by specialized cells: the *peptic* or chief cell, which forms the pepsin, and the *parietal* or oxyntic cell, which manufactures the hydrochloric acid.

THE "STOP" AND "GO" SIGNALS

What starts the complex secretory mechanism of the stomach going? First, it is probably never turned off completely. Day and night, even when we are not eating, even when we are sleeping, the secretory mechanism continues to work at very low levels in most individuals, much as the motor turns over while the car is idling in neutral gear. The stomach, as it were, is always prepared to digest a meal, ready in advance for whenever we will eat and supply it with food. Even before the meal itself arrives in the stomach, advance notice is sent to the stomach to start tuning up. This is the appetite juice—the sight, smell, and taste of food stimulates the stomach to prepare its juices. Even thoughts or dreams of food can turn on the stomach apparatus. This the brain does by switching on the vagus nerve, which runs from the head through the neck, alongside the esophagus to the stomach, and then sends impulses directly to the cells required to pour out acid and pepsin (the parietal and peptic cells already mentioned).

But the secretory engine really gets going when the meal arrives in the stomach. Just the mere stretching of the wall by the bulk of a meal sends local messages to the appropriate receiving stations on the parietal and chief cells. Even more important are the chemical signals, the breakdown products of protein, which act on a third stomach cell in the antrum (the antechamber I have already mentioned above)—the G-cell. The "G" stands for gastrin, a powerful hormone released directly into the blood which flows back to the stomach and stimulates the outpouring of acid. This accounts for about half of the acid secreted in response to a meal.

What about the stop signal? What gets the stomach back to neutral gear? As our appetite is satisfied, the appetite juice begins to slacken off as the vagus nerve stops sending its neural impulses directly from brain to stomach. Second, as the stomach has started emptying itself of both the solid and liquid parts of the meal, the pressure on its wall decreases. Thus the stretching or "distention" signals quiet down. Third, another intricately coordinated process comes into play. The acid secreted by the stomach runs over the G-cell in the antrum and turns off its chemical message. In this "feedback" process the stomach regulates itself like an automatic pilot or a thermostat.

Since Mother Nature or evolution leaves little to chance, when the contents of the stomach enter the upper gastrointestinal tract, acid and fatty products send messages back to the stomach to slow down. This signal is accomplished by the release of several hormones (the chemical messengers) from the duodenal lining cells.

The "start" and "stop" signals work in concert to adjust to the needs of the stomach and their own complex systems, producing just the right amount of stomach juice for that particular meal. Of course, these signals can get mixed and become a source of trouble.

Through the Alimentary Canal

So far we have traveled with the partially prepared meal from the mouth, through the esophagus, saw where it is ground fine by muscles of the stomach, and then emptied normally at a constant rate into the upper small intestine, the first portion of which is called the *duodenum*. It is in the small intestine—the long tube—that the major work of digestion takes place. *Digestion* is really the process in which the fats, starches, and proteins of our diet are broken down into their smaller components—amino acids, fatty acids, and simple sugars—and then absorbed.

The duodenum can be considered the meeting place of three roads. The main one comes from the stomach and is fed by two smaller pathways or ducts: the common bile duct that contributes the bile secreted by the liver, which is stored in the gallbladder, and the pancreatic duct adds the pancreatic enzymes which digest protein (trypsin and chymotrypsin) and fat (lipase), the starch-splitting enzyme (amylase), and an alkaline-containing bicarbonate in fluid form, so important for maintaining the proper chemical environment for these digestive ferments to work effectively (*Figure 3*). This bicarbonate-containing fluid—the body's antacid, as it were— also serves to neutralize the hydrochloric acid coming down from the stomach and thus prevents the duodenum from ulceration and inflammation. In addition to the pancreas, the lining in the duodenum also contributes soda bicarbonate to the mixture.

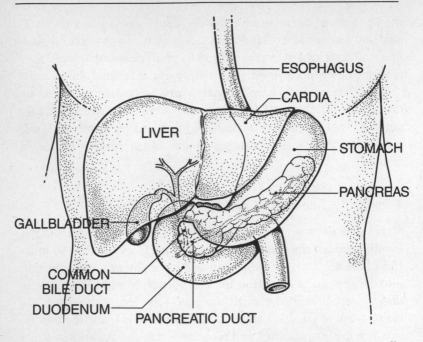

FIGURE 3. Details of the upper gastroduodenal area, including liver, gall-bladder, and pancreas.

"Stop" and "Go" Signals from the Duodenum

What sees to it that the pancreatic secretion of water and enzymes and the contribution of bile, so important for fat absorption, arrive in the duodenum just when they are needed there?

Just as in the stomach, neural impulses play a part while chemical messengers (hormones) play an even greater one. The presence of acid and some amino acids (products of the breakdown of protein) in the duodenum release two hormones into the blood. The first, *secretin,* sends a message to the pancreas to pour out water and bicarbonate and to the stomach to stop making acid. The second hormone, *cholecystokinin,* signals the pancreas to pour out and send along the three major groups of digestive enzymes and, at the same time, stimulates the gallbladder to contract and pass its bile down the common bile duct; simultaneously, this hormone relaxes the sphincter or "gatekeeper" at the lower end of the bile duct.

The Duodenum as the Guardian of the Small Bowel

From the duodenum, as we have observed, released chemical messages return to the stomach to slow down secretion and signal the gallbladder and pancreas to add their digestive enzymes to the meal, which is being moved along the long conveyor belt, the remainder of the small bowel. In addition, the duodenum sends messages on ahead, signaling the nerves and muscles to move the contents along by waves of muscular contractions, which we call *peristalsis*. Electrical signals in the wall of the duodenum—collectively called the *migrating motor complex* (MMC)—control this movement by activating the nerves and muscles downstream. The MMC, is the "housekeeper" of the duodenum, cleans out the corners and moves its contents along.

The lining of the duodenum can also sense local disturbances— an important point we return to when we discuss *nausea*. Messages are not only sent from the brain to the upper gut, but are sent from the upper gut to the brain. For this message service, the vagus nerve, already mentioned for its role in stimulating the stomach to secrete, contains thousands of fibers that transport signals back to the brain. The sensation of *nausea*, distressing in itself and often ending in vomiting, may arise from the first portion of the duodenum. Contraction of the duodenum, distending it with a balloon experimentally, and local inflammation or ulceration can lead to our feeling nauseated.

In the normal course of events, we receive little in the way of sensation from the small bowel, which is richly endowed with other nerve fibers that run along with the fibers of the autonomic (the automatic) sympathetic ganglia—except when something goes wrong. The major, indeed almost the only other, sensation we feel in the gut is that of pain. The chief trigger for this is muscular contraction. During an operation, the small bowel can be handled, even cut, without being sensed; but forceful contractions caused by mechanical blockage or irritation give rise to painful *cramps*.

Where and How Are the Parts of Our Diet Absorbed?

Almost all of the contents of our food and drink are absorbed in the small intestine after being broken down into their constituent parts. Here the fluids poured into the intestine by its own secretion are also absorbed back into the body. When the saliva, gastric acid secretion, bile, and pancreatic juice, plus fluid secreted by the intestinal cells, are added up, the resulting eight or nine quarts of water and salts are moved down the intestine daily. This large volume must be recaptured by the body or we would quickly become dehydrated and be required to drink huge amounts of water and other liquids constantly. Indeed, more than nine-tenths of this volume is reabsorbed in the lower portion of the intestine in the *ileum* (see *Figure 1*) in this recycling process, and only about one quart of liquid passes into the colon; even most of this liquid is avidly sucked back into the body, which is eager to hang onto all the water and salts that it can. As a result, only a small amount of water is lost into the normal stool.

So most of the salts—sodium, potassium, chloride, and bicarbonate—that result from digestion are reabsorbed by the body. But what of the *nutritional* part of our diet, including the necessary vitamins. In our diets fats furnish the majority of calories. One gram of fat yields nine calories; one gram of protein, four; and one gram of starch, four. Proteins furnish the building blocks of our body (amino acids) and carbohydrates (starches) give us the energy-yielding sugars. The fat-soluble vitamins—vitamins A, D, E, and K—move along with fats; the water-soluble ones—especially the B group—move along with the water content. Vitamin B12, so necessary for the manufacture of the red pigment of our blood hemoglobin, is part of a complex machinery. The B12 of our diet is joined

TABLE 1. Areas of Absorption

Duodenum	Iron and calcium absorbed
Jejunum	Protein, fat, sugars, water, minerals, electrolytes, salts, and vitamins (except B12) absorbed
Ileum	Salt, vitamin B12, and bile salts absorbed
Colon	Water and salts absorbed. Potassium secreted

by intrinsic factor, a substance secreted by the stomach, acted on by pancreatic enzymes, bound by calcium, and absorbed further down in the ileum by a special transfer mechanism.

When the *fats* are in their proper form—called *micelles* (a mixture of fatty acids surrounded by bile which acts like a detergent, very much like the soapy water we use to clean greasy dishes)—they are absorbed mainly in the jejunum. The *amino acids* of protein and the *simple sugar of starch* are absorbed along the entire small bowel. But the thirsty intestine is anxious not to lose the *bile salts;* they are brought back into the body by the ileum. Those bile salts that escape the recapture mechanism of the ileum and get into the colon may stimulate the lining to secrete water and thus act like the body's own cathartic (*Table 1*).

How Fast Do Our Meals Move Through the Upper Digestive Tract?

We all know how rapidly we chew our food and swallow it, often too fast, along with swallowed air as we talk and eat in animated conversation. The partially digested stomach contents begin to leave the stomach promptly, almost half of the meal has left by 90 minutes, almost all is gone by three hours, depending in part on its fat content.

The major portion of the meal going from the duodenum to the *cecum* (the first portion of the large bowel, the colon) moves at different speeds in different individuals. In some it can get there in 90 minutes or even a shorter time, in others the meal moves along at a slower pace, up to three or four hours. These variations in time have little meaning or consequence for our health.

The constituents of our diet, carbohydrates and proteins, are quickly absorbed from the jejunum; the fats take a bit longer. Diabetic individuals know that the sugar of a glass of orange juice can quickly correct the sensation of low blood sugar caused by insulin or other drugs. During the course of a regular mixed meal, the peak of our blood sugar is reached usually in one hour.

How Does Our Diet Get Across the Intestinal Lining into the Body?

This book is not intended to be a textbook on physiology, but it may be helpful to understand how things can go wrong during the process of digestion. In this discussion, we spend a little time on the machinery by which the body gets the contents of the intestinal tract across the gut wall into the body.

Fats

The fats of our diet, which give us a large part of our daily calorie intake, consist of long chains of fatty acids attached to glycerol—the so-called *triglycerides*. These fatty compounds do not dissolve in water; oil and water do not mix. They must be changed into a form that can be absorbed, and this is accomplished by a complex chemical rearrangement that takes place in the interior of the intestine. Here the triglycerides are split into their smaller components, the fatty acids, by the pancreatic fat-splitting enzymes (the lipases) and then coated by bile salts secreted by the liver. These transformed particles are the micelles which can now be transported across the intestinal cells. Once inside the cells of the intestinal lining, the fatty acids are put back together again to form triglycerides, but in a new form (the *chylomicrons*) suitable for transport into the blood and to all body tissues, where they are either used or stored as fats.

Carbohydrates

Carbohydrates—starches and sugars—are a major part of the calories of our diet. These sugars include lactose (the sugar of milk) and fructose (the sugar of fruit). Starch itself is made up of long chains of glucose, the major sugar of our blood and tissues. These long chains are split into shorter groups by the enzyme amylase, which is secreted by the salivary glands and the pancreas. The resultant combination of two molecules of sugar—the disaccharides, sucrose and lactose—are split even further by the enzymes sucrase and lactase into simple sugars (glucose, galactose, and fructose), which are then the proper shape and size for absorption by the lining cells of the small intestine. These simple sugars are carried by a specific carrier or transporter system that requires electrical and chemical processes to move the sugar into and across the intestinal cell and finally out the back door of the intestinal cell into the bloodstream.

Proteins

The proteins of our diet carry the building blocks of our tissues, the amino acids. To be absorbed, the protein must be split and released into amino acids. Protein digestion begins in the stomach with the pepsins, but continues in the duodenum with the work of the protein-splitting enzymes of the pancreas, a large family containing trypsin and chymotrypsin among others. The result of their action is to release mixtures of simple amino acids and duos or triplicates of amino acids (combinations of two or three amino acids). The single amino acids and the twins or triplets are carried across the gut by special conveyor belts that require electrical and chemical machinery. Once inside the cell wall, other enzymes split the twins and triplets into two or three separate amino acids, and all the singles are then transported into the portal circulation—the blood-carrying veins in the intestine which carry nutrition to the liver. Like the sugars, the amino acids enter by the front door facing the intestine lumen and leave by the back door facing the bloodstream.

This abbreviated account of a beautifully orchestrated process shows us how and where things could go wrong when we digest a simple meal. Any one of the many organs that contribute the necessary enzymes and secretions to this complex process can go awry and can wreak havoc. Aside from organ dysfunction, any disturbance in the surface lining cells of the intestine, by surgery or disease, can throw a monkey wrench into this necessary chain of events. Finally, a breakdown in the conveyor belt anywhere along the line obviously could and does create additional problems.

2

Indigestion and Dyspepsia, or the Stomach and Its Discontents

Getting the Words Right

You call it indigestion and you know what you mean: an unpleasant group of sensations and symptoms that seem somehow to arise from somewhere in your upper gut. These sensations include upper abdominal discomfort or pain, which is often felt below the breastbone as distention, a feeling of fullness, belching, bloating, nausea, even vomiting at times, and a feeling of filling up too quickly before you finish your meal. We doctors call it *dyspepsia* and we think we know what you mean.

Sometimes you use the word *heartburn* to mean a hot, burning, acid sensation just behind the breastbone, and we are sure we understand what is causing it. We can just imagine the acid in your stomach rising up into your esophagus. You can almost taste the acidity in your gullet and, on occasion, you may even get a mouth full of warm burning fluid, especially when bending over, and which may even waken you at night.

Often your indigestion keeps coming back and you are afraid you have or will soon develop an "ulcer," especially if you have been going through a period of great stress or have forgotten that you have been taking a lot of medicines for headaches or arthritic joint pain. The doctor, for his part, is afraid he may not be able to explain your problem or will have trouble sorting it out.

Then again, there is this thing we all call "gas." If you belch or burp up some air, your doctor knows what you are talking about. If you are flatulent and pass the gas through the rectum, it is clear what the patient is complaining about.

But very often you feel as if a balloon has been blown up inside your abdomen, you feel distended, your clothes feel tight over the abdomen, and it gets worse as the day goes on. Sometimes one even feels and hears gurgling sounds—air and liquid swirling around inside one's abdomen. We complain of gas, yet X-rays of the abdomen do not show air pockets or areas of the intestine filled with gas.

These problems of indigestion (dyspepsia) are important because they are so common. Perhaps as many as one-quarter of the population will complain of some of these kinds of symptoms over a six-month period. The time and cost of investigating these claims, as you can easily see, can become enormous.

Obviously we are not going to deal in this book with the occasional occurrence of these symptoms. You do not worry about them or consult a doctor if they occur only rarely. Most of us, I believe, tolerate these complaints for a short while. When they last for more than a month, or keep coming back, we then feel we need to get some relief and a diagnosis as well.

Sorting Out the Different Kinds of Indigestion

In thinking about the many different ways the normal functioning of the upper gastrointestinal tract can go wrong, it is useful to distinguish those due to organic medical conditions from those dyspepsias which do not appear to have an organic basis. In this book we will consider both in detail. Some are related to organic disease, peptic ulcer being the most important and most common, along with gallstones, pancreatitis (inflammation of the pancreas), growths of the stomach, and inflammation of the esophagus and stomach.

We must also deal with those conditions that do not have an organic basis, which, for lack of a better term, we will call the *functional group*. Do not make the assumption that, because we cannot easily locate an organic cause at present, these symptoms are neurotic or imaginary. The symptoms are real. You really are uncomfortable and suffer from bloating, distention, fullness, and belching, even if our ways of looking at the structure of the upper intestine with X-ray, or of looking directly into your stomach and duodenum, show no obvious structural abnormalities even with biopsies.

We are beginning to understand that the discomfort of indigestion may in fact arise from a disturbance in the muscular actions or activity of the esophagus, stomach, or duodenum. The problem is in the disturbance of those activities that move food and fluid along the giant conveyor belt of our digestive tract. The problem may be one of *motility*. Research and clinical investigations are just beginning to unravel the complex set of muscles and nerves, and their interaction, which moves the contents of the intestine along, and how these interactions can go wrong.

It is this group of functional indigestion or dyspepsias whose causes are subtle and, as yet, poorly understood—and, as such, make up the most interesting newer area of emerging information. Sometimes discoordinated and overactive muscular contractions give rise to pain and discomfort behind the breastbone and to spasm in the esophagus. At other times the stomach just simply cannot move its contents along and things back up.

Although your discomforts can overlap and can seem confusing, particular symptoms fit the profiles of distinct underlying disorders. For example, one associated with heartburn seems to point to the backup of the stomach's acid content—secretion plus food—into the esophagus.

Yet another group of symptoms may mimic what you have heard about peptic ulcers (hunger pains relieved by food or antacids); but no ulcer will be found on investigation. These kinds of symptoms are labeled non-ulcer dyspepsias.

A third group of complaints may center on the feeling that your stomach is just not emptying itself adequately. Food feels as though it is not leaving your stomach. You fill up quickly during a meal and are reluctant to continue eating. You have belching and burping, and the cause seems to be in the failure of the stomach and the muscles of the stomach wall. A mechanical failure of gastric contractions to empty the stomach seems to be at fault here.

At other times these upper intestinal symptoms seem to merge with lower abdominal ones—lower abdominal bloating and distention with irregularity of bowel movements. They suggest that the entire gastrointestinal tract is at fault, not merely the lower bowel, which points to the widely known *irritable bowel syndrome* (IBS).

In Chapter 4 we look at heartburn, its symptoms, causes, and effective treatments. In Chapter 5 we discuss and sort out ulcer dyspepsia from non-ulcer disease. The challenge for both the doctor and the patient is "getting the words right." From this collaboration your doctor can advise you of what forms of testing and treatment may be necessary.

3

Finding Out What Is Wrong

How Much Testing Must I Have?

When you consult your physician regarding the symptoms we lump together as "indigestion," how can he or she and you go about finding out the kind of difficulty you are experiencing—that is, how can we go about finding out the cause? Notice I have said the doctor and you, because this is a joint matter. The participation of the patient in the search is crucial. And without sounding overly optimistic, the search really does unravel much like a good detective story.

For your joint meeting on a group of complaints, write out a coherent story, if you can, beforehand or have some notes in an outline form. This will be a great help. When did these symptoms begin? Have they persisted unchanged or altered in any way? Is there a family history of this variety of troubles? Be sure to list any medicines you may have been taking recently or are still taking—including over-the-counter ones. It is easy to overlook aspirin-containing medicines, pills taken for premenstrual symptoms, all kinds of anti-arthritic drugs, and even the megadoses of vitamins.

The recent epidemic of the eosinophilia-myositis syndrome (now believed caused by the use of the amino acid, L-tryptophan, or a contaminant in its manufacture, taken to induce sleep) reminds us that we often forget that some preparations bought in health food stores may actually act as drugs as well as foods. The Omega III fatty acids derived from deep sea fish oils belong to the class of foods which have quite a few drug effects on the body's chemistry.

A simple list of your current eating habits will also be useful, including types of foods, time of meals, and skipped meals. Be candid about your habits regarding smoking, alcohol, and caffeine-containing beverages. Do not forget that cola drinks contain caffeine. Have you been on a liquid weight-reducing diet or a variety of fashionable fasting regimes? Are you taking Sorbitol-containing foods or candies in an effort to reduce your sugar intake? This kind of information may turn out to be unimportant, but you cannot predict its use to your physician. Be sure to express your own concern as to what these symptoms mean to you.

Usually after a general physical examination the question will arise as to what further studies and tests might need to be done. This general physical examination obviously will include a careful examination of the abdomen during which your doctor *inspects, listens* for abdominal noises and sounds with the stethoscope, *palpates* or feels for the normal organs (the liver, the spleen, the intestine, and the gallbladder), and *searches* for areas of tenderness, pain, or other abnormalities. The examination of the rectum with the finger—the digital rectal examination—is an obligatory part, in my opinion, of this physical examination. If any stool is present in the rectum, it should be tested then and there for evidence of blood, unless blood is obvious on the examining finger.

Two types of tests will then need to be considered, which we may label the *general* ones and then the more *specific gastrointestinal* ones. Since digestive symptoms may arise from nonintestinal disorders, some simple general tests are in the order: a blood count to rule out anemia or blood loss and some blood tests that can be used to assess kidney, thyroid, liver, and nutritional status.

The patient's need for information regarding the value and risks of the diagnostic tests arises once our physician tackles the specific question of indigestion. If the rectal examination yielded no stool or did not raise the question of bleeding, then of course most doctors would readily agree that a stool specimen is in order.

The search for hidden or occult blood in the stool is relatively easy today by using Hemoccult® cards. When I was a medical student, patients had the messy task of collecting their stools in a paper or glass container. Now, with the cards, the stools are passed into the toilet bowl and a portion fished out with a small stick, which accompanies the cards. A fragment of stool is then smeared onto a designated spot on the card. Most cards have places for two stool specimens. The card need not be fumigated, refrigerated, or kept under a glass bell jar, just mailed to your doctor. He need only add a drop or two of a chemical agent to the specimen spot and watch for a color change.

We may be put off at first when we realize that these specimens require careful collection, especially prior control of our diet, so we do not get a false positive or a false negative answer. A false positive test would result if the source of the blood in our stool were bleeding gums or the blood of the red meat we recently had eaten. A false negative test could arise if our stools really do contain blood, but the test does not reveal it because elements of our diet interfere with its detection. Such foods as horseradish or turnips or vitamin C tablets, for example, can contribute to a false negative result. So for three days before and during the collection periods, our diet needs to be carefully monitored—a nuisance, but so important.

So far we have been talking about painless, risk-free, and relatively inexpensive tests. Now we have to consider the more detailed tests commonly used for investigation of the upper gastrointestinal tract and its disorders. They fall into two main categories: *tests of structure* and *tests of the function*. The structural ones study the physical state of the organ—the parts as it were. The functional ones study the workings of these parts. A simple analogy may help to clarify this distinction: your auto does not start, the battery is dead and you need a new one, or the feed line is plugged and needs unclogging. These are *structural matters*. On the other hand, your new stereo system with all its modern equipment is producing noises, not music, from your brand-new cassettes; nothing appears to be wrong with the speakers or other equipment and so you decide that some fine tuning will do the trick. This is a *functional problem:* the *parts* of the apparatus are not working correctly.

Structural Tests: Checking the Structure of the Machinery

Esophagus and Stomach

We begin with tests of the *esophagus and stomach*. If your symptoms surround the act of swallowing or pain in the chest, and lung and heart trouble have been eliminated (not often easy to determine with regard to the heart), examination of the esophagus and stomach by X-ray using barium as the contrast medium—*the upper GI series (Figure 4)* as it is called—has been the standard method of studying these organs since the early years of the twentieth century. Of course, refinements in technique, with even the addition of videotape, have been added over the years. This method is without risk and we have permanent records of the shadows cast on film. It has proved its value beyond any doubt; however, it does not give us any direct pictures of how the tissues look and does not allow for the taking of biopsies of any suspicious areas or abnormalities.

The limitations of the upper GI series have been overcome by endoscopy, which permits the physician to view the gullet and stomach and even the upper small intestine and the duodenum with the *flexible endoscope,* which bends and allows light to be passed around curves. *Upper gastrointestinal endoscopy*—as this method is called—has become standardized, allows color pictures to be taken, is monitored by television techniques, and permits biopsies and cultures of tissue, as well as cultures for bacterial organisms or parasites, to be taken. The method has minimal discomfort with preliminary medication, entails considerable expense, and carries a small, but definite, risk of bleeding or perforation. But for many physicians, either in the office or hospital, it is the first approach to problems in this area. Each physician must decide, with the patient's

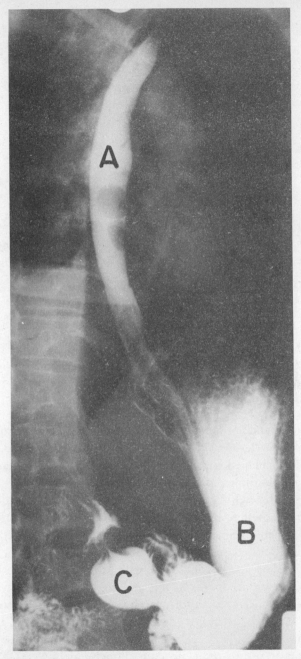

FIGURE 4. X-ray of the upper gastrointestinal tract visualized by a barium meal. A, esophagus; B, body of stomach; C, antrum of stomach.

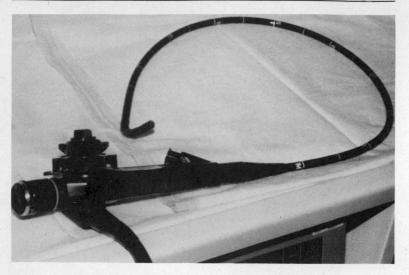

FIGURE 5. Photograph of upper gastrointestinal endoscope.

consent, which technique is needed for a particular person and problem (*Figure 5*).

Duodenum and Remainder of the Small Bowel

With X-rays and barium, the entire duodenum and the remainder of the small bowel—the *small bowel series*—can be viewed. Sometimes better detailed films of the small intestine can be obtained by putting the barium directly into the small intestine with a tube introduced through the mouth. This is the *enteroclysis* procedure, which has a definite but limited place. The upper gastrointestinal endoscope can display most of the duodenum. If the longer instrument used in the colon—the *colonoscope*—is employed, the viewer can get into the first portion of the jejunum. An even newer instrument—the *enteroscope*—can traverse the entire small bowel and view its whole length. Unfortunately, at present, this instrument cannot be used for biopsy or treatment—for example, to stop bleeding.

An important test of the structure of the small bowel is the *small bowel biopsy*. This is a biopsy of the lining cells of the duodenum and first portion of the jejunum. This test is done most often to see whether there is any inflammation or, more important, any loss or change in the lining cells to make the diagnosis of sprue or celiac disease in children, or better known in adults as *gluten enteropathy* (the result of an allergy to the protein gluten).

Gallbladder

The gallbladder can be imaged by X-ray using dyes which concentrate in that organ when given by mouth. This is the old-fashioned standard *oral cholecystogram*. This test is harmless and, except for people allergic to the iodine-containing dye, produces no significant reaction or effect, except for some diarrhea from the pills that are used.

More sensitive for the detection of gallbladder disease—especially stones—is the *sonogram or echogram*. It involves no radiation, only sound waves, and detects stones in about 95 to 98 percent of cases. The sonogram can also reveal whether the bile ducts are dilated or obstructed as well. At times, both the X-ray and the sonogram are used to give complementary information. In addition, we can use a radioactive labeled test called the *HIDA scan,* given intravenously, which will show whether or not dye can flow easily into the gallbladder. It is a good test of either obstruction of the outflow tract, the cystic duct of the gallbladder, or of acute inflammation of the gallbladder.

Liver and Pancreas

The size and shape of the liver can be seen on the *sonogram* and defects in the organ detected. This technique can also show us the diameter of the bile passage within the liver, evidences of blockage. The size and state of the liver as well as the spleen can be studied using a *liver and spleen scan* with the aid of an isotopically labeled material.

The pancreas can be outlined by the sonogram, as well as any defects in it, including swelling and stones. However, unlike the liver, viewing the pancreas can be difficult at times because of overlying intestinal gas.

The *computerized axial tomogram* (*CAT scan*) is a very sophisticated technique for visualizing the liver, gallbladder, and pancreas. This technique involves lying quietly on the X-ray table for at least 60 to 90 minutes. It is painless and without risk, except for those who cannot tolerate the intravenous contrast dye, which improves the quality of the study. Abdominal CAT scans, however, can be done without contrast matter if need be.

In this connection, a still newer method for imaging the abdominal organs is the nuclear *magnetic resonance imaging* (MRI) technique, which depends on magnetism, but no radiation. But cannot be used if there is any metal in the abdomen (for example, surgical clips or staples). For the abdominal organs, the CAT scan is often superior to the MRI, but both may occasionally be needed.

So far we have been discussing *noninvasive tests*. The important *invasive test* for diagnosing disorders of the pancreas and gallbladder and their ducts is the ERCP (*endoscopic retrograde cholangio-pancreatogram*—quite a mouthful). In this technique, a tube is passed through the mouth and stomach into the duodenum to the area where the bile and pancreatic ducts enter the duodenum. Contrast dye is injected in the ducts to determine the size and shape of the ducts and whether they are open (*Figure* 6).

The ERCP is not as uncomfortable as one might expect from this description. It gives valuable information which may not be obtained by other methods. The main risk is that, by injecting dye under pressure into the pancreas through the main pancreatic duct, one may stir up inflammation of the gland. This can occur in a few patients and usually subsides promptly. Unfortunately, the test, even in the hands of experts, may fail to show the duct one is especially interested in seeing.

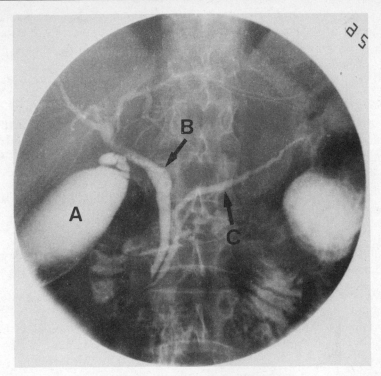

FIGURE 6. X-ray of endoscopic retrograde cholangiopancreatogram. A, gallbladder; B, common bile duct; C, main pancreatic duct.

Biopsies

LIVER AND PANCREAS

Sometimes it is crucial to biopsy the liver or pancreas—that is, obtain a fragment of the liver or pancreatic tissue for examination by the pathologist to make an accurate diagnosis of what is going on in these organs. This can be done nowadays with relative safety if the blood factors that control bleeding and blood coagulation are normal. It is performed by inserting a long, thin, "skinny" needle under local anesthesia through the skin of the abdomen. The needle's movement is guided by sonogram or CAT scan into the tissues of these two organs. In this way, the physician obtains a small piece of the organ for microscopic examination. This procedure is obviously one of the most invasive, but surprisingly enough causes little risk of serious injury to either gland or their surrounding tissues.

SMALL BOWEL

Sometimes, especially when we are investigating disorders of absorption, it is necessary to obtain a piece of the lining of the small intestine for microscopic examination. In this test, which sounds much worse than it really is, the patient swallows a capsule attached to a tube, which can obtain a fragment of the lining layer (the mucosal layer). If there are no defects in coagulation in the subject, this is a relatively safe procedure.

Functional Tests: Ways of Finding Out How Well the Parts Are Running

We now come to the functional tests that assess the working of this complex machinery.

Esophagus

To determine if the painful sensation the patient complains of comes from the esophagus, one can drip dilute hydrochloric acid through a tube into the esophagus to see if it reproduces the original pain. This—the *Bernstein test*—is useful in patients with inflammation of the esophagus.

If there is chest pain or difficulty in swallowing, then pressures can be measured in the upper and lower esophageal sphincters; the peristaltic waves in the body of the esophagus can also be recorded. This test—*esophageal manometry*—is most helpful when your physician is trying to sort out if your problem stems from how well things move through the esophagus, a problem of motility. This test requires the subject to swallow a soft, narrow, rubber tube which allows the pressure measurements to be recorded; it is essentially a risk-free procedure and not too unpleasant for the individual.

Devices are also available for finding out how often and how much stomach acid gets back into the esophagus; but, at present, these are cumbersome to use and are essentially research tools.

Stomach

We can gain useful information on how effectively the stomach moves food and fluid along by setting up a *gastric emptying scan,* since the stomach is better equipped to move food than barium. In this test, a subject is given a meal labeled with a radioisotope and a geiger counter is placed over the subject's abdomen to record the rate at which elements of the diet empty from the stomach into the duodenum. This gastric emptying scan is risk-free, painless, slightly tedious, and quite precise in detecting any meaningful delay in gastric emptying.

Other simple tests can tell us how much acid the stomach is secreting and can measure the blood level of the acid-stimulating hormone *gastrin* as well as *intrinsic factor,* which is needed for vitamin B12 absorption. In the past much emphasis was placed on the gastric analysis of acid in general; now its place has been better defined, and it is used infrequently at present.

Gallbladder

Simple blood studies will tell us if the bile passages are incompletely or completely blocked. When sonogram and X-ray studies fail to reveal the nature of the patient's problem, microscopic examination of bile, collected with a tube placed in the duodenum, can shed light on whether there are tiny stones or cholesterol crystals (which form stones). This is called *duodenal drainage.* This test too is almost risk-free and, when performed by those with experience, really not very unpleasant for the subject to take.

Another way of determining whether the gallbladder is functioning normally and whether the bile passages open enough to allow the free flow of bile is through the use of a HIDA scan. In this procedure, a dye labeled with radioisotopes, which can be tracked in the body, is given intravenously; then, at intervals, films are taken. This is especially useful in detecting the inflamed gallbladder, the condition known as *acute cholecystitis*.

Movement Through the Small Intestine

At times we need to find out how quickly or slowly material passes through the intestine. This can be done by taking X-rays at intervals after the subject drinks a liquid containing barium to see how long it takes the barium to reach the colon.

Tests of Absorption

Not only is it at times crucial to know how the small bowel looks on an X-ray, but to get some information on how well it is doing its job of *absorption*. I discuss disorders of malabsorption and maldigestion in Chapter 11. Here I only want to give the reader some idea of what information is available to answer these questions.

First, careful weight records are important. See if you can document your weight at specific times in the past.

Second, studies of the blood can measure your ability to absorb vitamin B12, folic acid, and iron, which are needed to make red blood cells and prevent anemia.

We are all familiar with the glucose tolerance test; this procedure measures the blood sugar after a dose of glucose by mouth and is usually performed to detect diabetes. For intestinal disorders we can measure lactose absorption—the sugar of milk—by the *oral lactose tolerance* test. We can obtain some measure of carbohydrate absorption—that is, other sugar absorption—by using the sugar *d-xylose* as a test substance. In this procedure, the five-hour output of d-xylose is measured in the urine after a specific dose by mouth; or the blood level may be determined. An abnormal d-xylose test usually indicates disturbances of the lining of the small intestine.

Fat absorption can be measured by collecting stools for 24, 48, or 72 hours while the subject is eating a diet rich in fat and then measuring how much fat escapes digestion and absorption by leaking into the stool. It can be a messy and unpleasant method, but an invaluable test at times. A simple test for excessive fat in the stool involves staining a smear of stool with a dye (Sudan Red) and examining it under the microscope to detect fat globules. This old-fashioned test, in my opinion, is not used enough these days before putting the patient through the more difficult and expensive one of collecting the entire stool output for a predetermined period of time.

Bacterial overgrowth of the small intestine by organisms, which ordinarily live in the colon and which migrate upstream to the small bowel, can be detected by breath tests that measure hydrogen released by bacteria in the small bowel which is then expired through the lungs.

How Much Testing Do You Really Need?

I have just presented you with a rather lengthy list of the kinds of tests and imaging techniques that tell us what is going on in the upper gastrointestinal tract. If we can pinpoint what might be the cause of your indigestion, we can begin to prescribe a treatment, perhaps even a new diet. But the question you really want to ask is "How much testing and how many more tests do I really need?" *In most instances, my answer is "Not very much" and "Not very many."*

For most people with indigestion, the important information comes from the careful and detailed story of your distress, followed by the general physical examination by your doctor—including the digital rectal examination plus some simple blood studies and examination of the stool. If the distress has been persistent, then, in most instances, pictures of the upper gastrointestinal tract (including the esophagus) or upper intestinal endoscopy, plus or minus the sonogram of the upper abdomen, may immediately solve the problem and lay the basis for treatment.

The more complex and invasive testing, of course, will be reserved by your physician for any important danger signal associated with your indigestion—such as bleeding, anemia, or weight loss.

On occasion, your doctor may suggest that your stool be examined for parasites or their eggs—called "ova"—when you complain of nausea or indigestion. This may seem rather peculiar to you since your complaints all seem to arise a long way from your lower bowel. But this examination may be quite informative, especially if there is any irregularity or looseness of your stools. The reason for this is the fact that the organism *Giardia lamblia* lives in the upper intestinal tract—especially in the duodenum—where the sensation of nausea often arises. *Giardia lamblia* has recently received lots of attention in the press. It seems to be everywhere, especially in water supplies, and various places around the world—such as Leningrad (now St. Petersburg), Aspen, and Zurmatt—have had epidemics of infestation of this organism.

Unfortunately, only about half of the time can they be found in the stools of those who carry them around. A repeat stool study can improve the score. If your doctor really suspects that this organism needs to be searched for thoroughly, then endoscopy of the duodenum through the mouth, with biopsy of the lining, is called for. Staining of duodenal secretions will have to be done to find this culprit.

ABCs Versus XYZs of Technology

I consider the history, a complete physical examination, rectal examination, blood and stool tests as the essential ABCs of the diagnosis. X-rays, sonogram, and endoscopic examination are midway between the ABCs and the XYZs of technology—the more complex techniques including CAT scan, MRI, biopsy, and ERCP.

There have been so many wonderful advances in our diagnostic technology that there is the tendency to skip some steps in the careful, safe, logical role of investigation and jump quickly to the more complex imaging techniques. This is not a plea for holistic medicine—whatever that may be! I want to emphasize that you and your physician ought to go over the advantages and risks—the drawbacks, if you will—of the proposed tests that may be needed to solve your problem.

Bear in mind that various standard tests are being improved all the time. For example, let's consider the use of barium. Remember that this substance is the contrast material used in standard X-rays of the gastrointestinal tract, but that the gastrointestinal tract was not designed to move barium along. Moreover, barium is heavier than water, so it may move by gravity alone. Food, on the other hand, does not move by gravity; it is moved along because of muscle contractions in the esophagus, stomach, and small bowel. To get information on how the stomach is emptying itself of real food, scans are obtained these days by labeling food and following its movement out of the stomach.

In this discussion, *functional* does not mean primarily psychogenic or stress-related problems. We will discuss these aspects of indigestion in Chapter 14. Here we have been interested in functional disorders that may occur at microscopic, biochemical, or even at electromicroscopic tissue levels.

Just as the electrocardiogram greatly advanced cardiology in the diagnosis and treatment of arrhythmias, so researchers are trying to perfect methods of measuring and recording the electrical activity of the small bowel and stomach. They are looking for a way of making these tests not only easy to perform, but easy to take! Moreover, the tests must be sensitive enough to detect disturbances of rhythm in that portion of the tract. This is an exciting chapter that is still unfolding.

II

SPECIFIC
PROBLEMS

4

Acid in the Gullet

Heartburn, Esophagitis, and Hiatal Hernia

Heartburn

If you have ever had the unpleasant sensation that its sufferers call "heartburn," you will know what we are talking about in this discussion. If you have never experienced it, you are indeed fortunate and rare, since most people have had it at some time in their lives and many women have it frequently during pregnancy. It is a burning discomfort felt in the chest just behind the breastbone, often ranging from the root of the neck to the lower end of the chest cage, with an occasional echo—as it were—in the corresponding area on the upper back of the chest. It may be, but need not be, accompanied by a sense or rush of highly acid fluid into the back of the throat with a very unpleasant stinging sensation there.

It is this retrosternal burning—that is, behind the sternum—that is the core of heartburn. And while the sufferer may have initial trouble swallowing, or even a pain in the front of the chest that may alarm him or her into thinking he or she is experiencing the prelude to a heart attack, these symptoms are not to be confused with angina.

41

Where and When Does This Discomfort Arise?

Heartburn arises in the esophagus and results from the presence of the stomach's acid contents in the lower end of the esophagus. The acid has a direct irritating effect because tissues there are not normally exposed and prepared for the acid and partially regurgitated material of the stomach. Physicians refer to this condition as *gastro-esophageal reflux*—the flowing backward of stomach contents into the esophagus. You will recall (from Chapter 1) that traffic through the esophagus from the mouth to the stomach is generally one-way, with the muscles propelling food downward and with the sphincter muscle at the lower end of the esophagus opening at the right time to allow material to pass through. In between swallows, this lower esophageal trap door remains usually closed, holding back reflux under most circumstances of normal swallowing.

From this brief description it is clear why heartburn is usually not present on awakening in the morning; the stomach is relatively empty at this time of day. Heartburn comes on regularly—if it does occur—after the stomach has been fed and stimulated to secrete acid and pepsin, which is needed for digesting a meal, and after the gastric muscles start contracting. Once this gastric machinery begins, the stage is set for heartburn. Since fluids do not flow uphill, you can understand why you might not have heartburn during the working day. But when you lie down to sleep at night or take a nap during the day, the contents of the stomach can more easily run back into the esophagus, especially if your stomach is full.

If the pressure in the esophagus exceeds the force that is keeping a lid on backward flow—the muscle power of the upper esophageal sphincter—then, of course, the refluxed contents would be regurgitated to the throat. If this material should spill over to the voice box and windpipe (the larynx and trachea), you would automatically cough in an effort to prevent yourself from choking or to clear this stuff out of your lung, or you might even become hoarse.

What Causes Heartburn?

The immediate cause is the acidity of the material refluxed into the lower end of the esophagus. The gastric acid—hydrochloric acid—directly irritates the surface layer of cells of the protective lining. This is easily proven by dripping dilute hydrochloric acid through the swallowing tube directly into the esophagus, thus reproducing the patient's heartburn and discomfort—the Bernstein test described in Chapter 3.

The normal concentration of acid from the stomach is strong enough and irritating enough to give you heartburn. Subjects with heartburn do not necessarily produce an overabundance of acid, as do some ulcer patients; they simply secrete normal amounts. If they secreted no acid at all, they would not have heartburn of this kind.

We have to go one step further to explain the cause of heartburn. It is not enough to have acid around in the contents of the stomach, it has to get into the esophagus. So we are back to the question: What causes reflux of gastric acid contents into the esophagus? We must remind ourselves of the many devices that nature has endowed the esophagus to protect itself.

When we swallow our saliva, we dilute the acid which is there and neutralize it so it is less irritating. If the muscles of the esophagus are not working appropriately in a coordinated fashion, they cannot sweep the acid out of the esophagus. Probably the most important protective device is the adequate functioning of the lower guardian of the esophagus, the lower esophageal sphincter. If this checkpoint, as it were, is defective and its pressure low, then gastric acid contents can sweep back across this unprotected frontier.

We must now turn to one of the major causes of the defective checkpoint—a hiatal hernia—on which we will spend some time.

What Is a Hiatal Hernia?

A hernia is simply a weakness of the abdominal muscle wall. We are all familiar with unbilical hernias (weaknesses in the area of the belly button) and inguinal hernias (weaknesses in the groin which allow abdominal contents to protrude). A hiatal hernia is simply a weakness of the diaphragm—the muscle which separates the abdominal cavity and its contents from the lungs. The diaphragmatic hiatal hernia is simply a weakness and widening of the aperture— the hiatus or opening in the diaphragm—that allows the esophagus to pass through the diaphragm from the chest cavity into the abdominal cavity. This weakness results in a protrusion of the stomach above the diaphragm, altering the angle at which the esophagus joins the stomach, weakening the ligaments that hold those organs together and in alignment, and most important impairing the lower esophageal sphincter's ability to prevent reflux.

What Else Affects Reflux?

The lower esophageal sphincter's pressure is reduced after a meal of fatty foods, by smoking, by the presence of acid in the stomach itself—all of which will favor reflux. Another important factor often overlooked, regarding reflux, is how successfully the stomach empties itself. It seems quite obvious that, if the stomach is slow in emptying or has difficulty in emptying itself, and it attempts nevertheless to move its contents on and finds the front door blocked, it will back them up out of the back door—in this case, the lower esophageal sphincter. This difficulty in gastric emptying can be caused by a mechanical blockage at the outlet—the pylorus— because of scarring from previous stomach ulcers in the channel or obstruction from a scarred duodenum due to an old healed duodenal ulcer.

At times the stomach may simply fail to have the necessary muscular strength to push its contents out. We call this *gastric paresis*. Frequently, diabetes is the cause of a prominent delay in gastric emptying. Other individuals, for unknown reasons or after a nondescript viral infection, may have a temporary delay in gastric emptying that lasts at times for months and disappears as mysteriously as it appeared. In some forms of heartburn, the stomach's ability to empty itself is one of several factors to be considered seriously by your physician.

How Much Testing Is Needed to Treat Heartburn?

Your detailed account of symptoms—how long you have had them and under what circumstances—is the most important clue to help your doctor make the diagnosis. A general physical examination, especially of the abdomen, and the rectal examination are essential in ruling out other diseases. The laboratory studies are quite simple: a blood count and a stool tested for hidden or occult bleeding are usually all that is needed. If there is no chest pain or difficulty in swallowing, an upper GI series with barium in the esophagus and stomach is in order if your heartburn has not already yielded to household remedies or over-the-counter antacids. It will help to establish whether any mechanical factor—such as a hiatal hernia—is contributing to the problem and whether there is evidence of old, new, or even silent ulcers of the esophagus, stomach, or duodenum. Also, the X-ray can furnish evidence of previous inflammation of the esophagus—esophagitis—with narrowing at any spot along the way and tell us whether the stomach is obstructed. While many physicians at present prefer to look down into the esophagus using the flexible upper gastro-intestinal endoscope, I would defer this form of imaging if this is the first time you are being investigated for heartburn, especially if your history does not suggest any complications or the need for biopsies.

In this connection, if there was any real suspicion that the stomach's failure to empty correctly is playing a part in your heartburn, it is useful to remember that the stomach was not designed to digest barium. Barium will leave the stomach promptly because it is heavier than water and has a high specific gravity, but food may not. This is important. The way in which food leaves the stomach can be measured with a gastric emptying scan after you have been given a meal—usually of scrambled eggs—labeled with a radioactive isotope. Its exit is observed under a geiger counter. There is no risk in either the upper GI series or the gastric emptying scan; both are painless, but boring.

How Should Heartburn Be Treated, and Why?

For some individuals, heartburn after an injudicious meal is such a commonplace occurrence, relieved by such over-the-counter pills as Tums®, that you may indeed wonder why the fuss. Avoid the meal, take a few antacid pills, and get on with your business.

The answer is simple and important: to prevent the development of the chronic inflammation of the esophagus known as *esophagitis*. We discuss the more serious problems—which can cause bleeding, pain, scarring, and difficulty in swallowing—in more detail in the sections on hiatal hernia and esophagitis in this chapter. Here it is enough to say that the chronic reflux of acid material into the lower end of the swallowing tube can cause a chronic condition with complications. *Prevention, rather than treatment of esophagitis, is the wiser course of action.*

I shall detail the care of heartburn by looking at your habits, diet, and lifestyle, and only then consider useful medications.

Treatment of heartburn and prevention of its complications are almost always medical, not surgical, procedures these days; and, if followed faithfully, are very effective.

Habits

Cigarette smoking is an irritant of the whole gastrointestinal tract; and with its disastrous effects on circulation, it clearly can retard ulcer healing. Smoking or sucking a cigar all day long can also lead to air swallowing—which increases stomach pressure and favors reflux. Smoking may relax the lower esophageal sphincter muscles by unknown effects.

Alcohol is an obvious insult to an already irritated lining of the esophagus by direct chemical injury.

Caffeine is such a large part of our diets that we are almost unaware of it. Coffee, tea, cocoa, chocolate, cola drinks with caffeine, medicines such as No-Doz®, or cold remedies containing caffeine or related compounds, are staples of American life. All these forms are powerful stimulants of gastric acids. Since you can get heartburn from normal amounts of acid in the stomach, you certainly do not need to add insult to injury by pouring out more hydrochloric acid. The moral is clear: If your heartburn is bothersome enough to consult a doctor or you are thinking of doing something about it medically, the big three—caffeine, alcohol, and cigarettes—must go. No easy matter!

Diet

We all agree that we should eat a healthy, well-balanced diet, rich in protein, low in animal fat, with lots of cereal grains, cooked vegetables, and fruit contributing their share of fiber. What about heartburn? Does food contribute? Common sense and a little reflection will remind us that certain highly seasoned dishes—different for each of us—have contributed to our heartburn. Heartburn does not mean ulcer. It does not mean eating unpalatable mush or goo for the rest of our lives. It does mean avoiding such highly spiced foods as delicatessen meats (pastrami or hot dogs), mustard, curry dishes, Szechuan cooking, and any number of other dishes. The list is as individual as each of us. Keeping the fats low also may help the sphincters to stay closed.

HOW YOU EAT IS JUST AS IMPORTANT

Skipping breakfast, skipping lunch, and then consuming a very large meal at the end of a tiring day certainly increases intragastric pressure and the possibility of reflux, especially if other factors, and stress, are already contributing to the problem. I have pointed out earlier that the likelihood of reflux is greater when an individual is lying down, with the stomach and esophagus horizontal, than when erect or sitting up. Since the stomach may take up to three or more hours to empty itself, it is obvious that you should not go to sleep or recline with a full stomach. Yet it is amazing how many otherwise sensible intelligent people do just that, though they are dimly aware there is something wrong in that habit. An easy rule to keep in mind: nothing by mouth after the evening meal and a decent interval before retiring—approximately three hours. All too often many of us end up on the couch, snacking all evening, and watching TV; however, if you want to avoid getting up in the middle of the night with heartburn, late-night nibbling will need to be eliminated. If you must put something into your mouth, remember fluids leave the stomach faster than solids. A cup of herbal or decaffeinated tea or decaffeinated coffee might be tolerated.

Medicines

The fundamental purpose of all medications used in treating heartburn is to reduce the acidity of the reflux material, clear the esophagus, strengthen the sphincter muscles, and help empty the stomach in a forward direction.

The acidity is lowered in two main ways. One is by *suppression* of the acidity in the stomach. The second is by *neutralization* of the acids already secreted.

To accomplish the first, we rely in great part on the class of substances called *histamine II blockers*. These drugs—Tagamet®, Zantac®, Pepcid®, and Axid®—act directly on the stomach's acid-secreting cell to stop it from making hydrochloric acid, especially during the long hours of the night when acid accumulates in the stomach and can reflux into the esophagus. More recently, a new class of anti-secretory antacid drugs have been developed. One, known chemically as Omeprazole and marketed formerly under the trade name Losec® (now Prilosec®), is a very powerful medicine that turns off the proton-pump—that is, the machine that secretes hydrochloric acid out of the manufacturing cell. We will be talking about this later in relation to the treatment of ulcer disease, but in general, it is felt that the patient should not stay on this for a long period of time.

For the second purpose—that is, neutralizing the acidity in the stomach—we use antacids in liquid form: for example, Maalox®, Mylanta®, Riopan®, Gelusil®, Amphogel®, or Alternagel®. These are given one and three hours after a meal in doses of one to two tablespoons and generally before sleep at night. To this group we may add over-the-counter antacid pills such as Tums® or Rolaids®.

To increase the esophagus's ability to clear itself of acid, strengthen the lower esophageal sphincter muscle's tome, and help gastric emptying, a number of medications are available. The oldest is a drug that mimics the action of the parasympathetic nervous system. Its generic name is bethanechol; its trade name is Urecholine®. More recently, we have come to depend on metoclopramide; its trade name is Reglan®. Sometimes the latter can cause unpleasant side effects of a neurological kind because metoclopramide crosses the blood-brain barrier. This can be overcome if need be by switching to another drug called domperidone—its trade name is Motilium®—which does not cross the blood-brain barrier. Domperidone, however, is not easily available in the United States, but can be obtained from abroad, especially Canada. These drugs are given in conjunction with meals, usually before them and especially on retiring at night. A third drug, the newest in our armamentarium, seems highly effective in emptying the stomach and does indeed increase the actions of the lower esophageal sphincter; it is known by the trade name of Cisapride®. Not available in the United States, except on an experimental and compassionate basis, it appears particularly effective with those whose reflux is due to delay in gastric emptying.

General Measures for Relieving Heartburn

Since reflux and its attendant heartburn often occur at night, sleeping with the chest elevated above the diaphragm will help prevent this distressing symptom. Placing a pillow under the chest, resting the head on two pillows, or elevating the head of the bed on blocks are useful maneuvers. A wedge under the mattress at its head is also helpful. All these measures need getting used to. You will need a footboard at the bottom of the bed to prevent your sliding down.

Trimming down, if overweight, avoiding constipation and its constant straining, and avoiding tight girdling or belts around the waist and abdomen are simple and sensible things to do.

Exercise

You may have wondered what bending, lifting, and bouncing around while exercising does to the reflux and acid. Recently, some studies compared the acidity in the esophagus in the fasting state and one hour after running, weight lifting, or bicycling. Running consistently caused the most reflux of acid. Weight lifting less so, and bicycling the least. I don't think you should choose your form of exercise by this test alone, but these are interesting findings. Exercise is probably of minor importance in causing the problem of heartburn, but terribly important of course for improving our general circulation.

Esophagitis

Now we need to explore a little further the condition of active inflammation of the esophagus—esophagitis—which is caused by persistent and chronic reflux of acid. It has been estimated that 10 percent of Americans suffer from chronic heartburn every day.

In addition to the burning sensation of heartburn, you may also complain of pain behind the breastbone spreading into the back or up into the neck, jaw, or even into the ears. This pain can be quite intense and frighten you into believing you are having a heart attack. Moreover, you may have trouble swallowing. Food seems to stick in your throat before going down the swallowing tube. The hot liquids you tolerated in the past, or even preferred, are now unpleasant to drink, and you experience distress as they are going down. You may have some nausea, but rarely vomit; on occasion, you feel you would be better off if you could. Being awakened at night with heartburn now is more frequent and annoying. You may have some acid fluid regurgitated into your throat causing you to cough. Sometimes you may even become hoarse, if the fluid spills over onto the vocal cords.

These symptoms are due to a more aggressive inflammation of the esophagus, which may even lead to bleeding. It rarely causes vomiting of blood, but blood might ooze from the inflamed surface of the esophagus and escape detection of the naked eye. This occult bleeding may cause the patient to become pale and anemic.

Do I Need Additional Tests for This Condition?

The X-rays of the esophagus and stomach (discussed earlier in this chapter) are clearly a must to determine whether there are any deep ulcerations of the lining of the esophagus, to see if you also have a peptic ulcer of the stomach or duodenum, to see if there is any mechanical narrowing as a result of previous inflammation and subsequent scarring, to diagnose a hiatal hernia—and especially to demonstrate whether the contents of the stomach (in this case, barium) can back up easily into the esophagus.

Another way of examining the esophagus and stomach is to look down directly into the esophagus with a flexible fiber-optic system—the upper gastrointestinal endoscope. This has become so widespread and relatively safe at present that often gastroenterologists, trained in its use, prefer to do this even without an X-ray. The endoscopic examination of the esophagus has the advantage of not using any radiation and allows clear, color pictures to be taken of the lining. It also permits the examiner to determine whether any narrowing is the result of a fixed scar or simply the result of spasm or inflammation. Most important, this technique allows biopsies to be taken of any surface area for study under the microscope by the pathologist. I prefer my patients to have an X-ray first as a roadmap for the endoscopist, since the test has a very slight—but definite— risk of complication, bleeding, or perforation. Its introduction, however, has been clearly a most important advance in the study of treatment of esophageal problems.

Methods for proving that an acid condition does exist within the esophagus or measuring the pressure of the esophagus at the lower sphincter ordinarily are not required at this stage of diagnosis or for planning the treatment.

Medical Treatment of Esophagitis

All the recommendations and suggestions listed earlier for the treatment of simple heartburn must be followed meticulously and vigorously for those suffering from esophagitis. Alcohol, smoking, and caffeine are absolutely forbidden. Other drugs, such as the non-steroidal anti-inflammatory drugs for arthritis (as well as aspirin), must be eliminated. The dietary suggestions of avoiding highly seasoned and fatty foods are to be followed rigorously. Elevating the chest above the abdomen (as discussed earlier) becomes even more important. All the medications—histamine II blockers to stop acidity, antacids, and drugs which may help to tighten the lower sphincter (Reglan®, Motilium®, Cisapride®)—must be used as well and consistently. Most important, the histamine II blockers (Tagamet®, Zantac®, Pepcid®, or Axid® in the appropriate doses) must be taken at bedtime and continued for a long time after all symptoms have cleared. Some have advocated a lifetime commitment to medication and a preventive course of action. Certainly, treatment for six months is worthwhile.

Clearly establishing and maintaining better eating habits seems to me a reasonable approach for the first attack. If the situation recurs, then medication should be continued indefinitely. The recent availability of Losec®, now known as Prilosec®, with FDA blessing, has made this powerful inhibitor of acid formation in the stomach an almost routine choice for use in esophagitis that is difficult to heal or persistent. How long it is reasonable or safe to continue to test this medication still remains an unanswered question.

Must I Have Surgery for Esophagitis?

Most patients today are treated medically and respond very nicely if they follow the prudent rules already outlined. If there is some mechanical blockage, narrowing, or scarring at the lower end of the esophagus, the medical program may also require dilating this narrowed section—some stretching of the narrow area—which can be done through the endoscopic tube by the passage of dilating tubes or balloons. Here the skillful therapist attempts to widen the aperture to allow easier swallowing and passage of diet and at the same time attempts to avoid too vigorous stretching which then would allow reflux to take place again in the future.

An Unusual Form of Esophagitis: Barrett's Esophagus

There is an unusual form of esophageal disorder which you ought to know about since your physician may tell you that you have a Barrett's esophagus when you consult him for what seems to be ordinary heartburn and the other symptoms of esophagitis. This is the condition named after the British surgeon N. R. Barrett.

Ordinarily, the esophagus is lined with a specific type of cell which resembles the skin, but in the presence of a hiatal hernia or in someone with a history of long-endured reflux or acid in the esophagus, this lining is altered in some few individuals. Now it resembles in part the cells along the upper portion of the stomach. This fact in itself is not important, but we have learned that this type of lining is more susceptible to cancer than might have been expected. There is no agreement at present about how often a patient should be examined with the endoscope and biopsied. My feeling, and it is only a feeling, is that this should be done about every one to two years. Vigorous medical treatment or surgical correction of reflux will often lead to a return of the normal cell lining, but whether this alters the suscepibility to cancer is unknown.

Hiatal Hernia

The demonstration of a *hiatal hernia*, which favors reflux of acid, often raises the question of surgery because hernias elsewhere— especially in the groin or inguinal area—are easily repaired by modern surgery. The basic point here is not the presence or absence of a hernia nor even how big it is (more about this later on), but whether it is involved in reflux. Is the hiatal hernia associated with malfunction of the normal antireflux machinery at the lower end of the sphincter? Hiatal hernia repair is not simply to put the stomach back below the diaphragm where it belongs, or to make the aperture in the diaphragm smaller; but to repair the antireflux mechanism so that it is effective again.

There are a variety of operations that have been shown to do the job. The details are not important here. The crucial question is when should they or do they need to be done. Clearly, simple heartburn or even esophagitis is not sufficient reason for an operation, especially since most patients improve with a careful medical program. Failure to respond medically after a conscientious trial raises the possibility of an operation and at this point should be taken more seriously. The complication of such recurrences—despite treatment—the development of strictures not responding to simple dilatation (*Bougienage* physicians call it), and the development, persistence, or recurrence of bleeding unresponsive to medical therapy are reasons for considering more aggressive procedures. Ordinarily, before such an operation is even a possibility, it must be demonstrated that you have reflux and, equally important, that the lower esophageal sphincter is defective. This necessitates the performance of esophageal pressure tests (see Chapter 3).

In this really not-unpleasant maneuver, the patient swallows a very thin, spaghetti-like tube which measures the pressure of the lower esophageal sphincter as recorded on an oscilloscope and moving tape. These pressure recordings, made in relation to swallowing, tell us whether or not the high-pressure zone at the lower end of the sphincter is present or is not working effectively. The tests will, therefore, also reveal whether the problem needs to be corrected surgically.

Operations for Hiatal Hernia

Operations for hiatal hernia to correct gastroesophageal reflux are serious, but not formidable, and require entering the left chest cavity as well as the abdomen. No organs are removed; they are merely put back into their proper place. Just as fashions change, so do the types of repairs of hiatal hernia for esophagitis change and vary from country to country, even within the Western world. I have the impression that I see fewer patients who have had, or are debating having, such operations these days. Perhaps our medical programs, which emphasize histamine II blocking agents and Prilosec®, now have made the difference. In the hands of a competent and experienced surgeon, hiatal hernia repair does the job very well.

There are two problems with the operation, however, that candidates for surgery should be aware of. Recurrence is one; and some difficulty in swallowing and bloating after surgery is the other. Hernias, wherever they occur, can recur after surgery, even in the best of hands; so it ought not to be surprising that an esophageal hiatal hernia can recur after an operation. But this is not frequent in my experience. Moreover, the job of making the sphincter muscles snug—which was the primary point of the operation—may have been done too well. The area may be too tightly sewed together, and patients have trouble swallowing or belching up air and feel distended and bloated.

While the difficulties in swallowing can be overcome by careful stretching of the esophagus, the risk is that the original looseness of that sphincter may recur. The inability to belch up a gas bubble from the stomach is annoying, but usually manageable in most instances without any instrumental attack on the repaired hiatal area.

Some Further Concern About Hiatal Hernias

So far we have been talking about hiatal hernias in relation to heartburn and to the development of esophagitis. But this weakness originating in the anatomical opening in the diaphragm deserves a little further consideration.

Hiatal hernias are common. Anything that increases the pressure within the abdomen can enlarge the diameter of the hiatus through which the lower end of the esophagus passes on its way to the stomach. Constipation with straining at stool, the fetus in the enlarging abdomen during pregnancy, tight abdominal binding from girdles, corsets, or belts, and abdominal obesity—all of these can contribute to the problem.

But as far as heartburn is concerned what is important is not how much of the stomach is pushed up under the chest above the diaphragm but how much the lower esophageal sphincter, the lower gatekeeper, is interfered with. As we have already discussed, the question is how much reflux of acid gastric content does the hernia allow?

However there is an additional question. Does the very presence of the stomach, or the upper part of it, above the diaphragm, cause trouble? If we are known to have a hiatal hernia, we have a tendency to blame any discomfort we experience at the lower end of the esophagus or the upper portion of our stomachs on this anatomical variation. In most instances the hernia is blamed unfairly. If the discomfort reaches a painful intensity, it is more likely that the pain arises from reasons, often gallbladder stones, other than the mere presence of the hernia.

But on rare occasions the stomach portion in the hernia can get caught or become twisted there temporarily; when the sufferer stands up, the stomach slips back into place. On even rarer occasions the pain persits because the portion of the upper stomach remains caught in the hernia. This pain is quite severe, may mimic a true heart attack, and may require surgical correction. This is most uncommon except in the even rarer condition, which is popularly called an *upside-down stomach*. In this situation the twisted stomach above the diaphragm is literally upside down.

More frequently a hiatal hernia can create problems in a subtle way by causing silent hidden bleeding, which is difficult to ferret out, or more drastically by causing the individual to vomit blood. Ordinarily tiny amounts of blood leak into the intestinal tract, but they are so small that they cannot be detected by our usual Hemoccult® test, cause no anemia, and have no importance. Even only one aspirin tablet a day will lead to a positive stool test, but this amount of blood lost daily does not cause any anemia or any clinical problem ordinarily.

The problems with hiatal hernia arise when an individual is either found to be anemic or to have occult (hidden) bleeding in the stool. Often our usual test by X-rays or endoscopy reveal no obvious cause for this bleeding except the presence of a hiatal hernia. This raises the question of whether small amounts of blood ooze from the lining layers of that portion of the stomach within the hernia, and whether this could be the site of the blood loss even if no gross ulceration is seen on looking through the endoscope. I believe this does occur in a number of instances, and I advise the same vigorous medical program that we have discussed earlier in this chapter for peptic esophagus.

On occasion an individual with a hiatal hernia may bleed more vigorously and then vomit blood. In this instance the source may be an acute ulcer which occurs just where the herniated portion of the stomach enters the neck of the hernia space. It seems as if the pressure at this portion of the ring of the hiatal hernia compresses the mucosa mechanically. This form of ulcer responds usually to standard ulcer therapy (discussed in the following chapter).

5

Peptic Ulcers

When the Stomach Digests Itself

In this chapter I want to talk about peptic ulcers, but a better term would be *peptic ulcer disease,* often abbreviated PUD.

I pointed out earlier that, while the process of digestion may begin in the mouth, really very little of our food is acted upon there. Transported rapidly through the esophagus (the swallowing tube), our meals have little time to be digested in that organ as well. The digestive process really begins in the stomach, where the pepsins—which are digestive enzymes or ferments—begin to break down the proteins we eat. These pepsins need to be in an acid bath to do their job. The stomach, as we all know, pours out acid as well as pepsin as needed. Indeed, even before the meal reaches the stomach, the specialized cells in the lining of the stomach wall have begun to secrete, stimulated by the thought, the smell, and the taste of an upcoming meal, in anticipation, of what will be needed next.

Why Doesn't the Stomach Digest Itself?

With such a well-developed machine for digesting our foodstuffs, you may well ask the question, "Why doesn't the stomach digest itself or its neighbor, the duodenum?"

The answer, of course, is that at times things do go wrong and the stomach can and does digest a part of its own lining or the lining of the duodenum. When it does, this local area of autodigestion leads to an ulcer on the surface of the organ's inner lining. The combination of acid and the enzyme, pepsin, is needed; these together do the damage. The resulting injury is called a *peptic ulcer*, which is essentially a localized, usually circular, loss of surface lining of the stomach or duodenum, rarely more than an inch in diameter.

How Does the Stomach Normally Protect Itself Against Damage from Acid and Pepsin?

Since there is usually a lot of acid and pepsin around, the stomach must take no chances. It has quite an effective defensive squad to handle the equally powerful offensive squad—to use a football metaphor. First, the surface lining cells pour forth a thick layer of mucus that coats the stomach wall like a layer of protective vaseline to keep the acid and liquid away. Second, the lining cells pour forth their own antacid, bicarbonate of soda, which can neutralize the acidity. Third, when acid approaches the surface lining, the surface cells seem to tighten up themselves and repel the acid. Finally, if injury takes place, neighboring surface cells rush in to fill the gaps and replace the damaged cells. If this were not enough, certain chemical substances in the lining—the prostaglandins—aid in the local defense work by increasing the nutrition locally, by increasing the blood flow to the troubled areas, and even increasing the amount of bicarbonate, antacid, and mucus. So you see that the stomach is a good machine to defend itself against autodigestion.

What Goes Wrong in the Individual with an Ulcer?

I have already said that the dirty work is done by the acid. The old slogan "no acid, no ulcer" still holds true since pepsin can only do its damage in the presence of acid. Therefore, you might suppose that the ulcer patient gets into trouble because he or she has too much acid. Yet this is not the case. Patients with stomach ulcers— that is, those with gastric ulcers—do not make more acid than normal individuals, and only a third of duodenal ulcer patients make excessive amounts of acid and so excessive acid cannot be the whole answer.

We must conclude at present that an ulcer develops when there is a breakdown in the balance between the offensive squad (the acid-pepsin attack) and the defensive squad (the normal protective machinery in the stomach wall).

Furthermore, we believe that the troubles more often are the result of local defenses rather than the aggressive acid-pepsin team. There is the rare situation in which the outpouring of acid is so great that no normal defensive mechanism can handle the flood of acid. This is known as the *Zollinger-Ellison syndrome,* often abbreviated as the Z-E syndrome. We shall talk about this later in the chapter. Weakness in the defensive apparatus, or weakness in the mucosal resistance, as we call it, is the culprit most of the time.

What Sets the Stage for Peptic Ulceration?

A number of factors can play their part in undermining the local defenses. Genetic factors must be involved since there are certain rare families who have an excessive number of individuals with peptic ulcer, but how the genes allow this is unknown.

Cigarette smoking has been repeatedly shown to impair ulcer healing and to favor an increase in the recurrence ulcers; but we do not know why. Many reasons have been proposed, including stimulation of acid formation, reduction in blood flow, increased reflux of bile from the duodenum into the stomach, or a reduction in the production of the prostaglandins. But whatever way cigarette smoking does its damage, the damage is clear. Psychological stress is also generally held by most individuals to play a part in starting an ulcer, but this is hard to prove. We all know hard-driving individuals in an organization who give ulcers rather than get them. Caffeine, a very strong chemical starter of acid secretion, has clearly been implicated, along with alcohol. While alcohol is not a strong stimulant of acid secretion, it can interfere with healing of the stomach lining. And, folklore suggests that spicy foods may play a part. While strong scientific evidence is hard to come by, one should not underestimate the possibility that such lore may contain bits of inherited wisdom.

Certain other diseases also seem to accompany peptic ulcers. Cirrhosis of the liver, secondary to alcohol, and chronic lung disease seem to be associated with more than their share of peptic ulcers.

Drugs and Ulcer Formation

The major point I want to make here is that aspirin is the chief example of a whole class of medicines that can injure the lining of the stomach and duodenum. This injury may vary from just surface irritation to ulceration and may even involve bleeding and perforation of these organs. This class of drugs is called the nonsteroidal, anti-inflammatory drugs (abbreviated NSAIDs) and are widely used for the treatment of many forms of arthritis as well as other muscle and joint pains. I spend more time discussing the important and potentially serious side effects of these drugs later in the chapter. Here I need only point out that NSAIDs seem to cause ulcers of two types. One is an ulcer out of the blue, so to speak, in individuals without any previous tendency to ulcer formation. The second is the development of an ulcer in those who suffer from an underlying tendency that makes them subject to more than their share of ulcers. These persons have a history of previous peptic ulcers, smoke cigarettes, and have been diagnosed as having illnesses related to alcohol.

A New Chapter in Our Understanding of Ulcers

The section you have just read on the factors that set the stage for peptic ulcers—the predisposing ones—represent, I believe, a fair summary of what has been thought and written about ulcer formation during the last 50 years. A new chapter, however, is being written, a chapter which is far from being completed, a chapter which is very hotly debated and eagerly being studied. The new idea is the intriguing concept that peptic ulcer may be due in part to an infectious agent!

A curious, curve-shaped bacillus has been seen in human stomachs for at least 100 years. Little, if any, attention was paid to this organism—now called *Helicobacter pylori* (abbreviated *H. pylori*) and formerly called *Campylobacter pyloridi*—until Bernard Marshall, an Australian investigator, and his co-worker, J. R. Warner, described its presence in human stomachs and associated it with gastritis, and its attendant inflammation of the lining, and with peptic ulcer. The association of gastritis of the stomach with duodenal ulcer has been known for a long time; but these investigators stressed the fact that a great many of these patients had *H. pylori* as well. In some studies up to 100 percent of patients with duodenal ulcer had *H. pylori* present. On the average, it was there in about 85 percent of patients with duodenal ulcer, somewhat less in gastric ulcer patients (about 65 percent had *H. pylori*).

The real problem is whether *H. pylori* causes the gastritis, the duodenal ulcer, and the gastric ones, or simply is a result of the inflammation and ulceration. This is no mere academic question. Obviously, if *H. pylori* is the cause, then its treatment and eradication should cure the ulcer condition. While the organism is a difficult one to get rid of, we do have medicines and combinations of medicines to help do the trick. Part of the problem is that *H. pylori* is in a large number of human stomachs. It is found in all human populations and increases as we get older—at about age 50 at least half of the individuals studied have the bacterium, even without having an ulcer or gastritis. So you may see that it is far from settled what *H. pylori* and ulcers have to do with each other. In the section on treatment of ulcers, I tell you what has been shown so far about treating ulcers by getting rid of *H. pylori*. For the moment, the scientific battle rages between those who stress acid as the main factor and those who incriminate the "bug"; still others have been trying to reconcile the gap between these two theories. In the meantime, there are a lot of patients with indigestion, even without ulcers, who are being treated as if the *H. pylori* were significant in their cases, even while the incidence of peptic ulcers seems to be falling.

How Do I Know if I Have an Ulcer?

We know now that the stomach and the first portion of the duodenum suffer bruises all the time with minor inflammation or erosions and even ulcers resulting from the ordinary wear and tear of eating, digesting, and living. Very often these ulcers are silent. They cause no distress unless a complication develops.

On the other hand, the upper gastrointestinal tract lets us know that there is a troublesome ulcer developing most often by discomfort felt high in the abdomen, in the mid-line, just below the rib cage and the breastbone. The discomfort can range from a mild ache—sometimes feeling like a hunger pang although you have just eaten—but at times the hunger pang can become more intense and become a true hunger pain. At other times the pain may be extreme and double us over. It may bore right through to the back. This is not heartburn, which results from acid backing up into the esophagus which does not cause an ulcer.

The striking feature of the pain of stomach and duodenal peptic ulcerations is the timing. The pain seems to come on after a meal—perhaps a half to one and a half to two hours after. It is temporarily relieved by eating again. You feel better with food in the stomach, since the food—especially its protein—acts as an antacid, neutralizing the acidity. Quite typically it lets us know it is there because we can be awakened with pain in the middle of the night, often from a sound sleep. This is clearly due to the fact that the stomach has emptied its last meal and is full of un-neutralized acid. Curiously enough, most patients with ulcer disease rarely have pain on awakening in the morning.

A lot of ingenuity has been devoted to trying to figure out what causes the ulcer pain. Probably the answer is twofold. Acid itself irritates the nerves at the base of the ulcer and muscular contractions or spasms also stimulate the inflamed nerves. Whatever the exact mechanism, sufferers soon learn that milk or any food or household remedies such as Tums®, Pepto-Bismol®, or over-the-counter antacids give relief, even if it is only temporary relief.

Nausea and vomiting may also signal us that an ulcer is developing. The duodenum is a very sensitive area of the gastrointestinal tract, and even the slightest disturbance there will cause nausea, which if strong enough can lead to vomiting.

Vomiting itself can call attention to the fact that the stomach is obstructed. The outlet is blocked because of some scars from previous ulcers near the outlet of the stomach. Most patients with obstructive ulcer have a pretty clear history of having had an ulcer for at least five years. Vomiting, often without pain, may be the only signal that they have been having ulcers on and off for a long time. Belching and burping are rarely signs of ulcer and are unjustly blamed on the gallbladder.

The Three Major Complications of Gastric and Duodenal Ulcer

The first important complication of ulcers is *obstruction*. I have already touched on it in the paragraph above. Since it is the result of scarring near the outlet of the stomach, it will lead to distention, bloating, nausea, and finally vomiting of the stomach contents. The obstruction need not be complete. The door may not be closed completely and tightly. Some material of our diet and stomach acids are moved along normally, but from time to time we may have quite painful vomiting. Obviously, in this case, appetite might fall off and nutritional needs will not be met. Equally important, and more immediately dangerous, however, is the resulting dehydration from the loss of water and the disturbance to the basic biochemistry of the body due to the loss of sodium and potassium electrolytes, as well as acid, from the stomach, with resulting leg cramps, prostration, and profound weakness.

A rarer complication that reveals the presence of an ulcer is *perforation*. The ulcer bores a hole in the wall of the stomach or duodenum and causes a sudden abdominal catastrophe of pain, shock, and hardening of the abdominal wall, which results from peritonitis. The hardening, often called *boardlike rigidity*, is easily recognized by the attending physician. This requires immediate medical and surgical attention.

Much more common is *bleeding* from an ulcer, which may be very slow and not easily detected or very rapid with the vomiting of blood from the mouth or the passage of blood through the rectum.

When blood is vomited from the stomach or duodenum in ulcer patients, the material looks like coffee grounds—a dark, brownish mess, rather than bright red. This is because the pigment of blood that gives it a red color is changed by the acid of the stomach into a brown pigment. When blood moves slowly through the intestine to exit into the stool, the red color is also changed and becomes a black, sticky mess. This is known as "tarry stool." It is not dark, but really black. Sometimes the bleeding may be so profuse that the blood has little time to be changed to color; in this case it will often appear bright red. Many people rarely look at the color of their stool, but they remember the advice on the Pepto-Bismol® package which points out that the bismuth contained in that medicine may give the stool a gray-slate color. This should not be confused with tarry stools. Sometimes the skin of tomatoes or blue- or blackberries may give the stool a reddish color or even a dark blue color. Again this must not be confused with true bleeding that can easily be detected by a simple color test in the office or now in sets available to the patient at home.

These complications are alarming, but you should remember that they are, fortunately, rare. Most often an ulcer remains silent during the life of an individual, except for pain after meals or at night.

How Is the Diagnosis of Peptic Ulcer Made?

The history of your complaints raises suspicion that you have or have had an ulcer. Let us begin with the simplest situation: you feel well in general, but you have the kind of pain that I have been describing and you have noted no change in the color of your stools. What needs to be done to be sure you do have an ulcer? In performing his or her physical examination, your doctor will check your weight and look at the color of your skin, lower eyelids, and nails to see if you are pale and may have lost some blood. In a simple peptic ulcer, the general physical examination may show only some tenderness over the area of pain when your abdomen is pressed upon. The rectal examination is in order to see the color of your stool and, if a fragment of stool can be obtained, it should be promptly examined and tested for the presence of blood by the simple colorometric test on prepared paper, the Hemoccult® test.

What Laboratory Studies and Tests Will You Need to Have?

Not too many, is the answer. A complete blood count is in order even if you have had no clear-cut evidence of bleeding to be sure you have not bled slowly without obvious blood in the stool. This form of bleeding is called "occult" or hidden bleeding. If, at the time of your first visit to the physician, no stool can be obtained and tested for blood, then you will need to use the special cards for the Hemoccult® test I have already described. Obviously, the dietary precautions must be adhered to, especially the one to avoid red meat.

I should say a word here about another special blood test which occasionally needs to be done. This blood test measures the levels of the hormone gastrin. You will recall in the section on the workings of the stomach that certain specialized cells in the antrum of the stomach secrete a chemical messenger, the hormone *gastrin,* that stimulates the acid cells to pour forth their liquid.

In ordinary peptic ulcer, especially duodenal ulcer, the level of gastrin in the blood is quite normal; but in the very rare condition of Zollinger-Ellison syndrome already mentioned, the gastrin levels are elevated. As promised, I spend a little time on this form of ulceration, which is most often associated with diarrhea, later in the chapter. However, with the common garden-variety ulcer, the test measuring blood gastrin level is not needed. In recurrences of ulcer, failure to respond to treatment or complications with the presence of diarrhea may raise the possibility of the Zollinger-Ellison syndrome.

How Is the Diagnosis Proved?

If your history is highly suggestive of peptic ulcer, your general physical examination is not remarkable, your blood count shows you are not anemic, and your stools are free of blood, what more, you may well ask, do you need? Why shouldn't your doctor simply treat you and make you feel better so that you can get on with your life?

The question is a very reasonable one. Many doctors would agree with you and start you on medication, postponing to see, locate, and record the ulcer only if you fail to get better or if you have a recurrence after responding for a while. My advice is different. I think that, whatever your age and however short or long your history, no matter how well you feel and look, we—your doctor and you—should be definite about the diagnosis and confirm it with reasonable and safe imaging tests for the following reasons:

1. Peptic ulcer, either gastric or duodenal, is a serious illness, not life-threatening perhaps, but with the risk of complications I have already mentioned.
2. The label is a serious one. Peptic ulcer has a tendency to recur and the tendency to be a lifetime one.
3. The diagnosis must inevitably involve the rearrangement of many aspects of your life, habits, and diet.
4. Present-day thinking in the field will lead to your taking medications for a long time, perhaps for some years, to prevent recurrences.
5. It will make a possible difference if you have a gastric stom-

ach ulcer rather than a duodenal ulcer. Duodenal ulcers are never malignant.

Differences Between Gastric and Duodenal Ulcers

Having said that duodenal peptic ulcers are never malignant, I now get quickly to the point of certain differences between gastric and duodenal ulcers, as well as similarities. For both, pain is similar with regard to location, timing, and response to food and antacids; but duodenal ulcers occur earlier in life, stomach ulcers later.

Both duodenal and gastric ulcers are associated with gastritis—that is, inflammation in the stomach. Duodenal ulcers are not malignant and never, as far as I know, become malignant. On the other hand, gastric ulcers may mask their seriousness and appear benign, but may indeed be cancerous. Even more disturbing is the fact that the pain associated with gastric cancer may respond to ulcer therapy temporarily and that these malignant ulcers act as if they are healing.

So you see we will continue to be anxious about leaving a gastric ulcerating lesion alone until we know it is benign and see that it heals completely. We want and expect all duodenal ulcers to heal and must take measures to be sure they do not recur; but we are haunted by the possibility of a gastric ulcer turning malignant or being malignant from the very beginning.

What Difference Does It Make if I Have a Gastric or Duodenal Ulcer?

The most important point I want to make here is that we have to be sure that your gastric ulcer is a benign one (duodenal ulcers are almost never cancerous). Gastric ulcers may mimic a cancer which is ulcerated, so at present every gastric ulcer should be seen through the endoscope and, more important, multiple biopsies taken of it to be certain that it is not malignant. While it is possible that a chronic, unhealed, gastric ulcer—after a long time—could become malignant, I doubt that this occurs except in rare instances. The ulcer is benign or malignant from the start, and several biopsies must be performed to be certain of the ulcer's status; however, failure to heal after a rigorous and long enough trial of medical therapy must raise the question of treating the ulcer with surgery. *You cannot walk around indefinitely, even if you feel well, with a raw unhealed ulcer in your stomach.*

Cancer aside, there is probably not much difference between gastric ulcers and duodenal ulcers, as far as treatment is concerned. Gastric ulcers probably need a longer course of therapy and more vigorous interventions, since they heal more slowly. Stomach ulcers that occur near the outlet of the stomach, in the pylorus, or antrum, behave more like duodenal ulcers. On the other hand, ulcers in the body of the stomach are often associated with *gastritis* and with lower secretion of acid (but there is some secretion). At present, it is believed that the organism *Helicobacter pylori* is found less frequently in gastric ulcer patients than in individuals with duodenal ulcers; but, as you already know, the exact role of this "bug" in all auspices is under intense study.

Imaging Techniques

So you can see why I believe every person suspected of an ulcer should have a permanent record and picture of his or her lesion. Until about fifteen years ago, the standard and safest way of diagnosing peptic ulcer was by X-ray. As I said earlier in Chapter 3, you would swallow the barium mixture by mouth, the radiologist would fluoroscope your stomach (that is, look at it under X-ray techniques), and then take permanent pictures of the lesion on the X-ray film. This is the upper GI series and probably remains the most frequently used technique. Its advantages include being well standardized, almost absolutely safe, and reasonable with regard to cost. Its limitations are clear too. It is a two-dimensional picture of a three-dimensional lesion, and no real-life color or appearance is recorded. It also fails to pick up very small lesions and has the most important limitation of being unable to give us any biopsies of the gastric ulcer or the stomach itself. Increasingly important these days, X-ray studies also cannot tell us whether the bacillus *H. pylori* is present, although a newer blood test can tell us whether you have been exposed to this organism.

Despite the limitations of the upper GI series that I have just listed, it still is a valuable method. It gives evidence on how the stomach and esophagus function as they move food along, discomfort is minimal, and a positive diagnosis of duodenal ulcer is definite and convincing.

The gastric ulceration presents more difficulties. Although the criteria for malignancy are well established, one may not be able to say unequivocally that a gastric lesion is benign by relying on an X-ray alone.

For this reason, the perfection of fiber optics—which allows light to be bent along flexible tubes—and the development of upper endoscopy represent a clear-cut breakthrough technique. In this method, after some local anesthesia has been applied to the throat and pharynx, a narrow tube—the fiber-optic endoscope—is passed through the mouth, down the esophagus, into the stomach and the first portion of the duodenum. The result is slight discomfort which is minimal in most instances. The technique allows the physician who does the tests to not only look at the lining but to photograph it in color and, more important, to biopsy it. This method also allows us to test whether the stomach contents or tissues reveal the presence of *H. pylori* if this is thought necessary.

Which tests should be done and in what order depends on the judgment, experience, and facility of your physician. I shall tell you my own view, my own bias, since I am one of the older generation of gastroenterologists who were not trained routinely to do endoscopy. My younger students learned this method from the first day they entered their training.

Although my conservative routine is to order an X-ray first, since I have access to extremely skilled expert radiologists, I agree with most gastroenterologists that endoscopy not only avoids radiation but gives excellent information. I use endoscopy for patients whose X-rays do not clearly reveal their problem, for those who fail to respond to treatment, or if there is any other discrepancy between the symptoms and the X-ray findings. The current trend is toward earlier endoscopy and even greater emphasis on the endoscope as the first, and only, imaging technique for studying patients with indigestion and possible ulcer. The same criterion holds true for endoscopy as with X-ray: the value of the test depends on the skill of the pair of eyes looking at the films or looking down at the image at the end of the tube.

Function Tests

X-rays and endoscopy tell us about the structure of the stomach and duodenum. Is there a place for tests of function that show us how well the organs are working? Years ago great emphasis was placed on measuring the exact degree of acidity in the stomach—by day or by night—in ulcer patients. Time has shown that they all have some acid in their stomachs. With the exception of those suffering from Z-E syndrome, it does not make any difference how much. So gastric analysis has fallen by the wayside.

Aside from imaging structure, X-rays tell us something about how the stomach empties. This is useful information if we suspect a delay or obstruction in emptying to explain your bloating, distention, nausea, or vomiting; but we must remember that the human stomach was not made to eat barium, but food. Barium, which is heavier than water, leaves the stomach by gravity. All other foods or fluids leave because of peristalsis or movement of the stomach muscles; so it is not difficult to understand that, when the patient may have delayed gastric emptying, it may not show up on a GI series. In this instance, he or she may need to have a gastric emptying scan using an isotopically labeled real meal (which I have described in Chapter 3).

The gastric emptying scan is rarely needed at the onset of an ulcer. It is only when individuals have repeated episodes of ulceration with healing and scarring that it may become necessary to prove their stomachs are partially or significantly obstructed. Complete obstruction is plainly shown by barium.

The Diagnosis Having Been Established, What Next?

What are our goals once the diagnosis is firm? You want prompt relief from the basic pain. Your doctor wants the ulcer to heal. You both want the ulcer to stay healed and not to come back. It will take a bit of doing to accomplish these goals. You will have to step back a bit with your physician and review your habits, your diet, your lifestyle, and our currently available list of medicines.

It should be reassuring that I have not mentioned surgery. In recent years with our newer medications, the need for surgery as a cure for ulcers that have failed to respond to current medical approaches has sharply plummeted. For complications, yes, surgery is recommended; for bleeding and obstruction, surgery becomes a clear and often necessary option. But for the common garden-variety ulcer, medicines alone will suffice in the vast majority of cases.

Diet

We are all aware of the cliché that "it is not what you eat, it is what is eating you." Although it is very hard to prove that diet rarely causes or even can cure peptic ulcer, you cannot help thinking that diet must make some difference in the healing of an ulcer. I share your instinct—even if we cannot prove it. Before your ulcer was firmly diagnosed, you probably tried to avoid highly seasoned or spicy foods, although you ordinarily enjoyed them.

In the absence of clear-cut scientific proof, it seems prudent to behave rationally. All will agree that we should eat a well-balanced nutritionally adequate diet, but beyond this, what else can one accept as reasonable? Avoiding highly acidic foods and drinks certainly is indicated if acid plays any role in ulcer disease, which we all agree it does to some degree. Indeed, most ulcer sufferers come to this conclusion themselves and have already cut out citrus fruits before they seek treatment. These fruits contain ascorbic acid (vitamin C) and ascetic acid. It would certainly be wise to avoid vinegar or dressings containing vinegar. *Bland* is a rather vague word, but it captures the need for a diet that is palatable enough to be eaten while not too appetizing to stimulate the gastric juices excessively. Remember that this is not a life sentence, but a reasonable approach to hasten healing.

Proteins are *amphoteric*—that is, they bind acids and alkalis. On the other hand, the products of their digestion—amino acids— stimulate stomach secretion. So a diet moderate in protein—fish, chicken, beef, egg whites—is probably in order.

Fiber—that is, the fiber of vegetables, salad, or fruit—raises a question mark for most individuals. Surely, our patients ask us, "With a sore in the stomach, won't fibrous foods cause injury or at least slow down healing?" The answer seems to be that there is no good evidence that this is so.

Fats and oil slow down and cut off acid secretion, so why not concentrate on them? Unfortunately, their effect on blood cholesterol—the high LDL fraction, the "bad" cholesterol—and their long-term harmful effects on the heart are still major reasons for all of us to avoid foods with high fat content, which most Americans still enjoy eating.

Milk has long been relied on by most laypersons as the ideal food for ulcers. Milk, by its volume as well as its chemical content, can dilute and neutralize acid. Certainly, low fat—that is, 1 to 2 percent—milk will avoid the possibility of too high a fat content in your diet. In the presence of normal kidneys, the high calcium content of milk and dairy products is perfectly safe; but I see no special virtue in a high milk intake for ulcer patients.

By cutting out citrus fruits and juices, we run the risk of reducing our vitamin C intake, but scurvy is not a real risk in most people's ulcer diets and can be prevented by a small amount of vitamin C in tablet form, which can leave the stomach quickly with a glass of water.

So in the end, we can add very little to the belief that diet does not play a major role in ulcer causation or healing. Obviously, having an ulcer does not have any effect on any known food intolerance we may have had in the past. You still must behave in keeping with your past dietary experiences, ulcer or not. Since we know that food can act as an antacid and give relief from pain, it follows that you should not skip meals or delay eating too long between meals. Since stretching the walls of the stomach can stimulate acid secretion, it is reasonable to have more frequent, smaller meals than fewer, large ones.

WHAT DO ACTUAL FOODSTUFFS DO TO ACID SECRETION?

You may very well think I have been walking around the subject of diet and peptic ulcer. Surely, you may ask: Have not researchers studied the effects of actual foodstuffs in the process of stimulating acid secretion?

This is quite a difficult job with humans, but it may be helpful and interesting to see how an animal stomach—quite similar in its working to ours—responds. The dog is an admirable animal for this type of research, at least in trying to determine the exact response to a given foodstuff. Dr. Charles F. Code and his co-workers at the Mayo Clinic, some 30 years ago, measured the acid response of about 24 foods in a specifically prepared dog's stomach. They found that the most gastric juice was formed within the first hour to hour and a half in most cases, but milk seemed to reach its peak of stimulation in the two to two-and-a-half-hour period after being drunk. Each food had its own characteristic response; rather similar patterns occurred within several distinct groups, such as bread and cheese; fruits and vegetables; milk and dairy products; meat, fish, and eggs. Protein produced the most acid. Starches, sugar, and fats produced the least.

As a group, meat, fish, and dairy products had the highest acid responses, while green peas, oatmeal, french fried potatoes, and some dried cereals the lowest. The foods producing the least amount from 100 calories were fruits (either raw or in juice form, preserved or fresh), butter, white bread, and dry cereal (corn flakes, for example).

This tells us what mostly happens in the process of acid secretion, but this explanation is somewhat artificial. After all, the foods themselves interact in the subject's stomach to create the acids; the complex environment of the stomach thus escapes clear observation. Equally important, our current research tells us little about how concentrated the acid is that drips into the duodenum to play its role in duodenal ulcer, or refluxes back into the esophagus to cause peptic esophagitis, or remains in the stomach during the long unprotected hours of the night. So the generalities I have already outlined in this section serve our purposes here and are the best interpretations we have of our findings to date.

Smoking, Caffeine, and Alcohol: The Big Three No-Nos

Here I will be dogmatic. Smoking, especially cigarette smoking, interferes with ulcer healing. The fact is rock hard. You must stop smoking if you wish to help your ulcer to heal and to stay healed. You know all the other important reasons for not smoking— ranging from avoiding cancer of the lung to protecting yourself against heart disease. In most respects I am a permissive parent, but I will not negotiate with you on the question of smoking. You must stop—cold turkey or with Smokenders®, hypnosis, whatever you wish or can, but you must stop.

Caffeine is a very strong stimulant of stomach acid, so caffeine-containing beverages and foods must also be avoided. Coffee, tea, and cola drinks contain caffeine, as do over-the-counter headache pills and pills to keep one awake. Actually, the list of such drugs is quite long (*Table 2*). In our society, we have all become accustomed to a large daily dose of caffeine. I make no rules forbidding caffeine in healthy individuals, but if you have an ulcer problem, caffeine is out.

Alcohol is not a strong stimulant of acid formation by the stomach. Yet you would not pour alcohol over a raw wound or ulceration without wincing. Alcohol is a local irritant and can damage tissues. I see no place for even moderate social drinking in a person with an active ulcer.

TABLE 2. Caffeine Content of Several Common Sources

Substance	Milligrams of caffeine
Coca-Cola (12 ounces)	46
Pepsi Cola (12 ounces)	38
No-Doz® (1 tablet)	100
Anacin® (1 tablet)	32
Excedrin® (1 tablet)	65
Decaffeinated coffee (6 ounces)	1–4
Percolated coffee (6 ounces)	40–175
Drip brewed coffee (6 ounces)	60–130
Instant coffee (6 ounces)	25–120
Brewed tea (6 ounces)	20–110
Instant tea (6 ounces)	25–50
Cocoa (6 ounces)	0–25

Ulcer Medication

The medicines we use to heal and prevent recurrence of peptic ulcers are of three main classes.

1. Antacids which neutralize the already formed acids in the stomach and duodenum.
2. Drugs which prevent the acid-secretory cell from making acid. These include the dramatic new group of histamine II blockers (which inlcude Cimetidine, Ranitidine, Famotidine, and Nizatidine), the drug Omeprazole marketed as Losec® and now as Prilosec® which acts directly and powerfully on the acid-making cell, and some other drugs which block neural impulses to the acid-secreting cell (these are called *anticholinergic drugs*).
3. Drugs which act to protect the lining of the stomach against damage, often called *cytoprotective drugs*. These include Sucralfate (Carafate®), which forms a viscous, sticky adherent gel, a protective layer as it were, over the normal injured tissues of the stomach and duodenum; and Misoprostol (marketed as Cytotec®), which shores up the lining tissues since it is a synthetic form of prostaglandin E1.

Until recently, most ulcers were treated with antacids and H-II blockers, but the current worldwide interest in the possibility that the bacterium *Helicobacter pylori* may play a role in ulcer formation and slow ulcer healing has revived interest in bismuth-containing medications, along with other antibiotics which are active agents against this organism (metronidazole [Flagyl®] and Amoxycillin®). Abroad much emphasis has been placed on a bismuth-containing compound, Bismuth Subcitrate (marketed as DeNol®), but this is not available as yet in the United States.

Antacids

Antacids have been used for time immemorial to relieve the pain of ulcers. For a long time, soda bicarb (sodium bicarbonate) was the antacid most frequently taken by patients. During the last 50 years, the gels have become the most popular, among them are aluminum hydroxide, magnesium hydroxide, calcium carbonate, and aluminum phosphate. And for some time it was thought that these agents only relieve pain; now we know that they hasten healing if given in large enough doses for a long enough period. Most ulcers will heal in 12 weeks.

Since soda bicarb is absorbed into the body and disturbs the acid-base balance of the blood and tissues, as well as the functioning of our kidneys, especially if given along with the ritual use of milk rich in calcium, this absorbable antacid is no longer recommended and should not be used.

The other antacids are called nonabsorbable antacids because they remain in the intestine where they neutralize the acidity. These agents vary among themselves and differ with respect to their effect on the bowels, their sodium or salt content, their neutralizing ability for a given-size tablet, liquid dose, or tablet antacid, and their cost (*Table 3*). The aluminum compounds—the hydroxide and the phosphate—may cause constipation and are often combined with agents to loosen the stool, especially magnesium hydroxide. The sodium content—which many individuals, especially those with high blood pressure, must watch—varies tremendously from prod-

TABLE 3. Some Tablet and Liquid Antacids

Composition	Brand Name	Sodium content (mg/tablet)
TABLET ANTACIDS		
Aluminum hydroxide, magnesium hydroxide	Camalox®	1.5
Aluminum hydroxide	Amphogel®	7.0
Aluminum carbonate	Rolaids®	53.0
Aluminum hydroxide, magnesium hydroxide, simethicone	Maalox Plus®	1.4
	Mylanta II®	1.1
	Gelusil II®	2.1
	Riopan Plus®	0.3
Calcium carbonate	Tums®	2.7
Calcium carbonate, glycine	Titralac®	0.3
LIQUID ANTACIDS		
Aluminum hydroxide, magnesium hydroxide	Maalox TC®	1.2
Aluminum hydroxide, magnesium hydroxide, simethicone	Maalox Plus®	2.5
	Mylanta II®	1.1
	Gelusil®	0.7
	Gelusil II®	1.3
	Riopan Plus®	0.7
Calcium carbonate, glycine	Titralac®	11.0

uct to product. You must take this into account if you are on a low sodium diet for any reason whatsoever. The use of simethicone for its antibubble or antigas effect is probably of little importance, but it is used in a large number of the commercially available and popular forms of antacid.

Liquid forms of antacid work more quickly than the tablet form and may have an advantage in speed and relief. Whether they are more effective in healing in the long run has not been proved.

Table 3 lists the chemical and trade names of a variety of liquid and tablet antacids and their sodium content. Their effects are similar, but they taste differently, affect the bowels differently, and vary in cost.

HOW MUCH ANTACID MUST I TAKE TO RELIEVE MY PAIN AND HEAL MY ULCER, AND FOR HOW LONG?

While there has been much debate over the amount of antacid one should take, at present the general consensus is as follows. You ought to take one ounce (30 cc) or one tablet of the double-strength antacid (such as Mylanta II® or Maalox TC®) twice after each of your three daily meals—meaning one hour after eating and three hours after eating—as well as at bedtime for a total of seven doses of antacid der day. This ritual should be followed for four weeks.

CAN I GET INTO TROUBLE WITH LARGE AMOUNTS OF ANTACID?

There are few dangers in the antacid treatment of your ulcer. If there is any problem in the working of your kidneys, the magnesium-containing antacids should be avoided. Antacids containing calcium, magnesium, and aluminum may interfere with the absorption of the antibiotic tetracycline and the absorption of iron and Cimetidine (Tagamet®). The major point to emphasize here is that relief of pain takes place very quickly with antacids long before the ulcer is completely healed, so you must stay with your program for at least four weeks.

Histamine II Blockers

Since the introduction of this class of drugs in 1977, we have seen dramatic results in our treatment of patients with ulcers—gastric and duodenal. At present, unlike antacids, these drugs are capable of actually blocking the formation of acid by the stomach. They include four drugs—Cimetidine (Tagamet®), Ranitidine (Zantac®), Famotidine (Pepcid®), Nizatidine (Axid®)—all of which act directly on the mechanisms within the acid-forming cells of the stomach lining to reduce the acid, almost but not completely.

In divided doses or in a single dose at bedtime, they appear to be equally effective in their results, and no one form has any great advantage over the others. Taken for four weeks, all can heal about 85 to 90 percent of ulcers, with gastric ulcers requiring a longer treatment period than duodenal ones. *Table 4* gives some current *suggested* doses of these drugs for gastric and duodenal ulcers. While a very small percentage of individuals taking these pills may have some reversible side effects, they are a remarkably safe group, enjoy tremendous popularity throughout the world, and probably are the most prescribed class of medicines in the world today.

The side effects may be different with each compound. Cimetidine is associated with swelling of the male breast in a small number of individuals and some mental confusion was thought to occur in the elderly. I have observed neither of these. Some patients receiving Cimetidine along with other drugs may need to have the doses of these drugs reduced to prevent excessive effects. These drugs include theophylline for asthma, warfarin, an anticoagulant (known as Coumadin®), an anticonvulsive drug Diazepam, which is a tranquilizer, and certain cardiac drugs (lidocaine, propranolol, and procainamide).

WHY DO SOME ULCER PATIENTS FAIL TO HEAL, EVEN WITH THESE POWERFUL AND DRAMATIC MEDICATIONS?

Since the prescribed program with these drugs is quite simple and may even be reduced to just one pill at bedtime, failure to follow the physician's suggestions is rarely the reason an ulcer fails to heal. In

TABLE 4. Histamine II–Blocking Drugs for Ulcer Disease

	Climetidine	*Ranitidine*	*Famotidine*	*Nizatidine*
Brand name	Tagamet®	Zantac®	Pepcid®	Axid®
Duodenal ulcer				
Active	800 mg qhs	150 mg bid	20 mg bid	150 mg bid
To heal	400 mg bid	300 mg qhs	40 mg qhs	300 mg qhs
Maintenance				
To prevent recurrence	400 mg qhs	150 mg qhs	20 mg qhs	150 mg qhs
Gastric ulcer				
Active	300 mg bid	150 mg bid		

mg = Milligrams.
qhs = At bedtime.
bid = Twice daily.

my experience, a strong family history of ulcer, onset at an early age, continuous use of alcohol, and, more serious, the continued use of cigarettes seem to be the most important factors for these individuals' difficulties.

Failure to respond to a careful program of histamine II blockers and antacids raises the suspicion that perhaps *H. pylori* might also be involved and needs to be eradicated, but this has yet to be proved, although recent evidence points in this direction.

IF MY ULCER HEALS AND I AM WELL, HOW LONG DO I REMAIN ON THE HISTAMINE II BLOCKERS?

I have not discussed maintenance therapy in the previous section on antacids because it is just not feasible to expect that you will be taking doses of antacid indefinitely. The question of whether to take the histamine II blockers prophylactically—to maintain healing—is quite different. One pill at bedtime is a quite reasonable approach. The basic facts are clear. Peptic ulcers tend to recur quite rapidly after treatment has stopped. The old slogan was "once an ulcer, always an ulcer!"

When we are talking now about recurrence of ulcers, we are speaking of ulcers that cause symptoms. Remember that ulcers may recur and be seen endoscopically even when you are not having any discomfort. We certainly are not going to use endoscopy on everyone with an ulcer who is quite comfortable.

If you consider only symptomatic ulcers—those that are causing abdominal pain and discomfort—there is good evidence now that the four histamine II blockers will reduce the recurrence rate significantly, perhaps as low as 30 to 35 percent. This clearly is a therapeutic gain worth taking advantage of. Since some of these studies have been done for more than six years, I doubt the improvement is different with any one of these compounds. I suggest you stay with the histamine II blocker that worked for you.

WILL THESE DRUGS CONTINUE TO PROTECT?

While some recent evidence suggests that certain doses of these medications will result in the suppression of slightly less acid with time, there is no reason to worry about their failure to continue healing.

CAN THIS SUPPRESSION OF ACID DO ME ANY HARM?

This question deserves some thought. We know acid and pepsin can be absent in the digestive process without any harm as, for example, in patients with vitamin B12 deficiency or in people who have had their stomach removed by surgery. Something else, however, may be very important; that is, the disinfectant activity of acid in the upper intestine. And yet people taking H-II blockers for long periods do not seem to have more intestinal infection than others who do not. Finally, these drugs do not abolish acid completely. We discuss the risks of complete loss of acid over time when we deal with the Omeprazole group of drugs later in this chapter.

Anticholinergic Drugs

For many years before the synthesis of the histamine II blockers, we relied on antacids plus some drugs that block the impulses that descend from the brain to the stomach by way of the vagus nerve. Pro-Banthine® was the best known of these drugs affecting the neural pathways, and some more recent forms are still available. This class of drugs suppressed acid secretion, but did not abolish it completely. The side effects were troublesome and occasionally injurious. They dried up secretions in the mouth, resulting in difficulty in chewing, tasting, and swallowing. Occasionally, they blurred vision and, most important, interfered with men's urination if they had any problems with their prostate. Understandably, these drugs have fallen into disuse. However, modest doses of Pro-Banthine® (7.5 and 15 mg) can be helpful at times, especially when they slow gastric emptying and thus allow longer times for antacids to stay in the stomach and to neutralize its acid contents more completely.

Cytoprotective Drugs

This class of medicines helps ulcers heal, not by affecting the formation of acid, but by protecting the lining of the stomach and especially the ulcer itself against further injury. In other words, they increase the lining's defensive forces.

Sucralfate (marketed as Carafate®) has been approved for use in the United States since 1981. It is a combination of sucrose and polyaluminum hydroxide which, in the stomach, forms a viscous adhesive gel-like cover that binds to the normal mucosa; in fact, it sticks even more tenaciously to erosions and the base of ulcerations for at least six hours after a dose by mouth. Carafate® does nothing to acid secretion; instead, it binds and renders inactive the enzyme pepsin and protects the ulcer base from being attacked by acid, pepsin, or bile. This drug comes in one-gram tablets and is taken either one hour before or two hours after a meal and at bedtime for a total of four grams. Two tablets twice daily have been shown to heal duodenal ulcers and relieve symptoms, and are as effective as the histamine II blockers, both for inducing healing and protecting the patient against recurrences. The same holds true for gastric ulcers, but as usual gastric ulcers are harder to heal and drugs require a longer time to work than in the case of duodenal ulcers. Sucralfate has few side effects, the most common of which is constipation. It can also interfere with the absorption of a number of medicines, including tetracycline, Cimetidine, Dilantin®, Digoxin®, and Coumadin®; it should not be taken within two hours of taking these drugs.

Misoprostol is the other cytoprotective agent now available in the United States. As pointed out earlier, it is a synthetic form of prostaglandin E1 that protects the stomach in a number of ways. With high doses, it cuts down acid secretion and protects the lining against injury by several routes, including stimulating the stomach to put out more mucus and bicarbonate, which naturally neutralizes acidity. Marketed as Cytotec®, in 100- or 200-mg tablets, it has been approved to protect the stomach against aspirin and other nonsteroidal, anti-inflammatory drugs, which are discussed in greater detail later in this chapter. In its ability to safeguard the lining, it is probably more effective than other current ulcer drugs. Side effects are not very common, except for diarrhea in some patients. It is reported to be effective with both gastric and duodenal ulcers, but in ulcers that form as a result of causes other than drug ingestion, its place is far from established. Its role in the maintenance therapy of gastric and duodenal ulcers has also not yet been shown.

Omeprazole

The search for better and better medicines to stop the stomach from secreting any acid is a lively one. The drug Omeprazole was marketed under the trade name of Losec®, and has been changed to the name Prilosec®, so as not to be confused with the drug Lasix®. Prilosec® has been available in the United States since October 1989 and represents the most powerful drug of this type yet developed. It works by stopping the pump that pushes hydrochloric acid out of the parietal cell (the acid-forming cell). The appropriate doses can stop the stomach from making any acid for at least 24 hours; but it has its effect only on the stomach. Since it is so effective, it can probably heal gastric and duodenal ulcers faster than the H-II blockers, with one tablet (20 mg) taken daily for four weeks.

If this is the case, why don't we all switch to Omeprazole immediately? Why has the Food and Drug Administration restricted its indefinite use, except in patients with the Zollinger-Ellison syndrome? Moreover, the FDA has restricted its use for the treatment of peptic esophagitis for periods of 12 weeks.

WHAT LIMITS OMEPRAZOLE'S USE?

When the stomach no longer makes acid, the acid-damper on the G-cell of the antrum (see Chapter 1) is removed. With the decrease in stomach acid, increased amounts of the hormone gastrin are produced to stimulate acid secretion. Since the stomach cannot make any acid on Omeprazole, it should give us no alarm, despite the turning on of the gastrin-secreting cell.

BUT THERE IS A CATCH

The elevated blood levels of the hormone gastrin can stimulate another type of cell in the antrum—the enterochromaffin-like cell (ECL)—whose exact function is not clear. In rats given ten times the human dose of Omeprazole for two years, gastrin released by Omeprazole led to a low-grade tumor of the antrum (carcinoid-like, they are called). No such tumor has been reported in humans who have take Omeprazole, but this finding has restricted the continous, unlimited use of the drug to patients with the Z-E syndrome.

The Zollinger-Ellison Syndrome

I have mentioned Zollinger-Ellison syndrome (Z-E) several times so we should at least here discuss this unusual form of ulcer disease. It is the only form of ulcer disease that is clearly related to the fact that the subjects secrete very large amounts of almost pure hydrochloric acid and the ulcer is the result of this agent alone. When the acid secretion is blocked, the ulcer heals. The problem is the excessive amount of acid. The condition is caused by the one mechanism that stimulates acid secretion in this case—that is, by the increased amount of the hormone gastrin in the blood that drives the acid cells continuously at a very high speed. This hypergastrinemia in the blood results from a small tumor of the G or gastrin cell—an adenoma. The tumor (often called a *gastrinoma*) may be single or exist in a number of places, often in the pancreas or duodenum or in tissues around the stomach or spleen. In this chapter, devoted to peptic ulcer in general, we need not spend much time on the way we search for this slow-growing tumor, but you should know that patients with the Z-E syndrome secrete so much acid they have diarrhea—which is rarely present in the garden-variety peptic ulcer. Skilled physicians will suspect the presence of this disease, and the gastrin level in the blood is easily measured today with a readily available test.

Should every patient with a peptic ulcer have a blood gastrin test? Probably not, unless there is something peculiar about the symptoms reported or the treatment—for example, failure to respond, prompt relapse after responding, or complications of the ulcer. These problems should prompt your physician to search for a gastrin-secreting tumor. Omeprazole is the drug of choice for this condition, which should be continued indefinitely.

Bismuth

For years patients and doctors have used bismuth for a variety of digestive difficulties. In the United States, bismuth subsalicylate (Pepto-Bismol®) has been available over the counter for the treatment of indigestion and diarrhea. Another form of bismuth, bismuth subcitrate (marketed in Britain as DeNol®), has been shown to be effective in treating duodenal ulcers, probably as effectively as all current histamine II blockers.

Now suddenly with the new research on the infectious bacterium *Helicobacter pylori* and its possible role in causing peptic ulcers, the role of bismuth and other antibiotics is a very intense area of investigation since these drugs can attack the organism directly.

The basic problem with this research is that the exact role of *H. pylori* in gastric and duodenal ulcers has not yet been established. The organism is present in almost every stomach, and it is quite difficult to get rid of completely. Nevertheless, combinations of bismuth (such as Pepto-Bismol® or DeNol®) and antibiotics (such as metronidazole [that is, Flagyl®] and Amoxicillin®) can eliminate the organism if used long enough. The claim has been made that the recurrence of ulcers may be the result of *H. pylori*'s presence. Some ulcers that are difficult to heal may need to have the organism eliminated.

For the time being, an ordinary peptic ulcer which responds to antisecretory drugs does not need tests for *H. pylori*. If the ulcer recurs promptly or is stubborn in healing, however, one should consider looking for *H. pylori*. This means fiberoptic endoscopy or the upper GI tract with biopsies of tissues and cultures to detect the organism. Blood tests to demonstrate the presence of the organism by measuring an antibody to *H. pylori* are now available for routine bedside use.

A WORD ABOUT THE SAFETY OF BISMUTH

Since the commonest form of bismuth used in the United States is bismuth subsalicylate, it is reassuring to know that the blood levels of bismuth and salicylate reached with the usual prescribed doses are considered safe in recent studies and are far below those considered toxic. The same seems to be true for the subcitrate form of bismuth widely used outside the United States for the treatment of peptic ulcers.

Drug-Related Peptic Ulcers

Earlier, when we discussed how the stomach and the upper intestine protect themselves against local injury that may lead to ulcers, you will recall that in the battle the defenses of the lining cells played an important part. The secretion of a protective coating of mucus—a sticky, gel-like coating—and the formation of an alkaline antacid substance (bicarbonate of soda) were the main defenses against the digestive acid and pepsin assaults. Equally important is the ability of the local tissues to repair the small surface injuries and erosions that occur daily in the course of ordinary eating. These local defensive measures are carried out by a group of substances called *prostaglandins,* which play a part in the mucosal defense apparatus. These substances also reduce the amount of acid the stomach is producing throughout the day. Unfortunately, aspirin and the entire group of drugs used for the treatment of arthritis can cause serious ulcerations of the stomach and duodenum by interfering with the synthesis of prostaglandins. *Nonsteroidal, anti-inflammatory drugs* is the label given to these medicines (frequently abbreviated as NSAIDs; *Tables 5* and 6).

We all take aspirin and NSAIDs for headaches or cold symptoms, and frequently do without any trouble. However, if we have a history of ulcer disease—with or without complications—our doctors will generally warn us about the risk of having side effects, such as heartburn (dyspepsia) or the possibility of stirring up an old ulcer or even its complications, especially bleeding.

Nowadays many of us are taking aspirin, sometimes baby aspirin tablets, daily or every other day to prevent clots forming in the blood vessels of our hearts or brains, especially if we have had a heart attack. Although this may not give us any intestinal symptoms, it can lead to obvious bleeding if you have or have had an ulcer. And it can lead to the unexpected finding of hidden—or occult—blood in our stools when they are routinely examined during our periodic health checkups.

But even more important and dangerous is the fact that people suffering from chronic arthritis—whether the wear-and-tear arthritis known as *osteoarthritis* or the more disabling *rheumatoid arthritis*—must and do take NSAIDs for long periods of time, even years. The evidence is quite clear that serious gastrointestinal problems, such as ulceration, bleeding, and perforation, can occur in patients taking NSAIDs—without warning or any minor upper intestinal discomfort or indigestion. This is so widespread that the FDA has insisted that warnings and information about the possible side effects be included in the package inserts for these medicines.

TABLE 5. Nonsteroidal Anti-inflammatory Drugs (NSAIDs)

Manufacturer	Generic name	Trade name
Bristol-Myers	Ibuprofen	Nuprin®
Ciba-Geigy	Diclofenac sodium	Voltaren®
	Phenylbutazone	Butazolidin®
Dista	Fenoprofen calcium	Nalfon®
McNeil	Tolmetin sodium	Tolectin®
Merck Sharp & Dohme	Diflunisal	Dolobid®
	Indomethacin	Indocin®
	Sulindac	Clinoril®
Parke-Davis	Meclofenamate sodium	Meclomen®
	Mefenamic acid	Ponstel®
Pfizer	Piroxicam	Feldene®
Syntex	Naproxen	Naprosyn®
	Naproxen sodium	Anaprox®
Upjohn	Flurbiprofen	Ansaid®
	Ibuprofen	Motrin®
Whitehall	Ibuprofen	Advil®
Wyeth-Ayerst	Ketoprofen	Orudis®

TABLE 6. Partial List of Medications with Aspirin or Aspirinlike Substances

Alka-Seltzer®	Darvon Compound®	Percogesic®
A.P.C.	Dristan®	Pabirin Buffered Tabs®
Ascodeen-30®	Duragesic®	Robaxisal®
Ascriptin®	Ecotrin®	Sine-Off®
Aspirin	Empirin®	SK-65 Compound®
Aspirin suppositories	Equagesic®	Stero-Darvon with A.S.A.®
Bufferin®	Excedrin®	Supac®
Cama-Inley Tabs®	Fiorinal®	Synalogos®
Congespirin®	Midol®	Vanquish®
Coricidin®	Norgesic®	

Note: All these substances have the potential to inflame or ulcerate the upper and lower gastrointestinal tract.

HOW OFTEN DO PATIENTS GET INTO TROUBLE FROM NSAIDs USED FOR ARTHRITIS?

In studies in which people took these NSAID drugs for several months to two years, difficulties occurred in about 1 percent of patients who used them from three to six months and in about 2 to 4 percent of patients who used them for one year. So we can readily appreciate this is no trivial problem.

WHO IS MORE AT RISK FOR GETTING THESE SERIOUS COMPLICATIONS?

Except for those with a history of peptic ulcer and such risk factors as alcoholism or smoking, no special group of patients stand out as targets. But we know elderly patients and those with debilitating illnesses tolerate bleeding, ulceration, and perforation less well than others. This is especially true in patients with rheumatoid arthritis. Whether other drugs taken at the same time—such as steroids or cortisone—contribute to ulceration is not known, but the larger the dose of NSAIDs, the greater the risk. Current belief is that there is no difference between the various drugs themselves or combinations of them.

HOW CAN ONE PREVENT ULCERATIONS FROM NSAIDs?

The drugs usually used in the treatment of stomach and duodenal ulcers—the histamine II blockers (Tagamet®, Zantac®, Pepcid®, Axid®), Sucralfate, or antacids—do not seem to prevent this form of ulceration even if taken regularly to protect the stomach. More encouraging is a recent discovery that prostaglandins—in the form of a synthetic prostaglandin, Misoprostol—markedly reduce the development of stomach ulcers in patients with osteoarthritis. Not enough is now known about whether this form of treatment, commerically available as Cytotec®, works in preventing duodenal ulcers.

SO WHAT SHOULD ONE DO?

Obviously, the first step is to discuss with your doctor the risks to you of these drugs and to consider other forms of treatment that may be less risky, perhaps accepting some symptoms as the price for freedom from the risks of a more serious disease. Second, try to get by with the smallest dose and the shortest period of continuous treatment. Finally, your doctor may advise Misoprostol as a continuous preventive treatment and monitor your long-term use of the drug as more information becomes available. My own approach would be to try to get the NSAID drug out of one's stomach quickly since it does most (but not all) of its damage there. A large glass of water will certainly help in this regard. Since antacids contain aluminum and medicines containing bismuth stimulate the stomach cells to secrete prostaglandin, I would take them even if it has not been proved scientifically that they help. They can do little harm if taken judiciously. If I were to have to take NSAIDs for a long time, I certainly would investigate Misoprostol.

IF I DO GET A STOMACH ULCER OR DUODENAL ULCER FROM THESE DRUGS, WHAT CAN BE DONE?

You must stop using the drug. Most of the common remedies for ulcers work, but they may take a longer time than usual. The newer prostaglandin analogue, Cytotec®, works.

WHAT TO DO IF YOU MUST REMAIN ON NSAID

If you have had a life-threatening complication—massive bleeding or perforation—I think you should never return to these drugs. Furthermore, we really do not know the best way to treat the NSAID-induced ulceration. If you must or elect to remain on these drugs, I myself would take antacids and histamine II blockers (such as Tagamet®, Zantac®, Pepcid®, Axid®) and use Misoprostol if further reports show it to be harmless for extended use.

Other Drugs and Substances that Injure the Stomach and Upper Intestine

I have spent a great deal of time discussing nonsteroidal anti-inflammatory drugs because they are used so frequently, so widely, and for such long periods that many individuals give them little thought. However, other drugs and substances can also injure the gastrointestinal lining.

In normal individuals, alcohol injures the stomach lining by causing erosion, swelling, and inflammation. For those who have had a peptic ulcer, alcohol use may stir up an old problem. It does this probably by breaking down the local protective machinery I have already discussed, and not usually by increasing the acidity of the stomach, as many might think. (Interestingly enough, beer, which is 5 percent alcohol, and wine, which contains up to 12 percent alcohol, can increase acidity; but whiskey, even diluted to 10 percent, does not.) The damage that alcohol does is increased when aspirin or other nonsteroidal, anti-inflammatory drugs are taken along with the alcoholic drink.

Tobacco, discussed earlier in connection with its role in slowing the healing process in ulcer patients, can induce chronic inflammation of the stomach—chronic gastritis—and clearly contributes to the symptoms of dyspepsia or indigestion itself. And we all know that cigarette smoking and the drinking of caffeinated beverages often go hand-in-hand (or "cup-in-hand"), as do cigarettes and alcohol, so it is hard to separate the distinct ill effects of each.

Caffeine is present in much of our daily environment and routine—in coffee, tea, soft drinks of the cola variety, chocolate, and cocoa; in drugs for migraines and headaches; and in over-the-counter stimulants to keep us awake, such as No-Doz®. In normal animals, caffeine was shown to damage the lining of the stomach. In humans it causes a powerful secretion of acid. In fact, caffeine was once used as a test substance to see if patients could secrete acid, and how much.

In light of what we do know and without being fanatical about it, I believe that caffeine can contribute to gastric irritation and in some people may give rise to indigestion. Since milk or cream will reduce the acid effects of caffeine, perhaps this is a help for those who must have that "morning lift" to get started on the day's tasks.

Steroids (*Cortisone*)

With so much discussion about the nonsteroidal drugs, what about steroid (cortisone-containing) medication? The matter is far from settled. Large doses seem to aggravate known duodenal or stomach ulcers and possibly do stir up old ones as well. Whether they can cause injury to the normal stomach and go on to produce gastritis with symptoms—even ulcer and perforation—has been hotly debated in the past. My own opinion is that steroids can, in some instances, induce stomach and duodenal trouble; I cannot, however, predict those who will get into trouble. I have no evidence that any medication will prevent this from happening, so I do not routinely give histamine II blockers to patients receiving short- or long-term steroids for their other disorders. I can even remember studies which reported to show that steroids could heal ulcers, but I would not count on that. On the other hand, it is quite routine for some physicians to give the histamine II blockers to patients receiving prednisone, especially in those who are going to use the drug for long periods of time, which would be the case with Crohn's disease and ulcerative colitis.

Bugs and Drugs

Earlier sections of this chapter reported our discovery of the bacterium *Helicobacter pylori* and devoted some space to our insights on what role this organism might play in peptic ulcer disease. Still to be explored is the possibility that this organism might play a corresponding role in the formation, and thus in the treatment, of inflammation, which has already been associated with the NSAIDs group. This opportunistic organism is known for its ability to find a vulnerable area to invade and colonize. We do not know if or how the bugs and the drugs interact, or whether *H. pylori* in a normal stomach increases the chances of NSAIDs causing troubles. In patients with known duodenal or gastric ulcer, one cannot help feeling that *H. pylori* is doing no good and should be eliminated if ulceration persists or recurs.

The Stomach After Surgery

Over the last few years, the number of patients being operated on for either ulcer disease or peptic esophagitis due to a hiatal hernia has decreased greatly because of our widespread use of the acid-stopping drugs we have been talking about in this chapter.

Yet people did undergo surgery in the past, and some still do, to control their ulcer disease and its complications in the esophagus, stomach, or duodenum. Unfortunately, some patients have a new and persistent set of symptoms after surgery which can be very annoying to them and disappointing to their physicians.

Almost all ulcer operations today interrupt or cut the vagus nerve to the stomach to reduce in some way the secretion of acid, but the severing of the vagus (*vagotomy*) interferes with the smooth emptying of the stomach. Individuals may have either rapid emptying of liquid and semisolid meals or quite the opposite—a delay in emptying, the *gastroparesis* we have discussed already. What is frustrating is that the symptoms for both rapid emptying and delay in emptying may be quite similar: sense of fullness, nausea, possibly even vomiting, general indigestion, and dyspepsia. Once X-ray and endoscopic studies have ruled out the possibility that the original ulcer disease has recurred, a gastric emptying scan is important in trying to separate the slow from the fast stomachs.

After a conventional operation for reflux disease of the esophagus, *fundoplication,* fullness after eating and bloating may develop. These symptoms, too, are blamed on damage to the vagus nerve during the operation, although this may very well not be the whole story. Digestive disturbances with the emptying of solid foods have been observed in some of these patients as well.

In any case, treatment of the postoperative stomach is difficult. As I have mentioned, separating the delayed from the accelerated emptiers is essential. For stomachs that delay in emptying, patients should take frequent, small, low-fat meals along with prokinetic medications (Reglan®, Motilium®, Cisapride®) in an effort to avoid further surgery, which may require removal of a portion of the second half of the stomach.

For stomachs that empty too quickly, patients should eat small, frequent meals and stop the use of free sugars—that is, sugar from the sugar bowl, candies, and concentrated sweets. Sometimes the antiserotonin drug cyproheptadine (Periactin®) may help with symptoms such as palpitation, sweating, and feelings of faintness.

Bloating in the patient after an operation for hiatal hernia is even more difficult to help. If food gets stuck or slowed down near the junction of the esophagus and stomach, the too-tight opening will have to be dilated by balloons passed through the esophagus. Again, this stretching needs to be done quite expertly since one does not want to open the door too widely and again set the stage for reflux! There is a place for the stimulating drugs—the prokinetic ones—in this not-too-rare complication of hiatal hernia surgery.

6

Non-Ulcer Dyspepsia

Indigestion Without a Label

You complain to your physician, "I am having trouble with my stomach." You feel uncomfortable and point to your upper abdomen. Your distress is halfway between discomfort and pain. It is not really heartburn you are complaining about, and yet it verges on that symptom. You do not feel very sick. Indeed, you feel rather well in general; but you feel something is gnawing high in your intestinal tract. Sometimes you experience a slight sense of nausea, but you never vomit. You are not sure whether eating helps or not. The household remedies you have tried—such as Pepto-Bismol®, Tums®, or Rolaids®—give you uncertain relief.

These uncomfortable upper abdominal symptoms seem to come on after eating, but you have no trouble swallowing food, and swallowing causes no discomfort. Occasionally, the discomfort comes on during the meal, but more frequently afterward, within a half-hour to an hour or two. You feel full in the upper abdomen and your body seems to be telling you that something is not working right.

These common symptoms usually are accompanied by more than a sense of fullness. You feel your upper abdomen is distended, swollen. A tight bra or tight belt needs to be loosened for you to get comfortable. We have all experienced these symptoms of indigestion (*dyspepsia,* as we physicians label it) from time to time; but when they return more and more persistently and annoyingly, then we consult our doctors—fearful that we have or are developing an ulcer. This combination of uncomfortable symptoms can be very mild or may increase in intensity and be uncomfortable, even painful. The nausea, for example, may get quite intense and even lead to vomiting. When our discomfort after eating comes on so regularly, it will not be long before we become reluctant to eat and even lose weight—further increasing our anxiety that we are developing a serious digestive problem.

Often these dyspeptic discomforts turn out to have no easily found cause or have no discernible organic basis. This combination of symptoms without an organic label is among the most frequent for which doctors and gastroenterologists are consulted. Only the functional symptoms we label *irritable bowel syndrome* are reported more often and purportedly are the most common reason a patient seeks the help of a gastrointestinal specialist. Just as the irritable bowel syndrome (IBS) can mimic a variety of other lower abdominal and colonic disorders and so becomes a diagnosis arrived at by process of elimination, so too the non-ulcer or upper abdominal dyspeptic symptoms can mimic a host of other digestive ailments. The overlap of this form of indigestion with other upper intestinal diseases means that an important part of the diagnostic problem would be to eliminate any serious organic possibilities.

How Is the Diagnosis Established?

As always, the most important preliminary test is a careful history of your difficulties. A good appetite, no disturbance of weight, no obvious disturbance in basic bowel pattern, and lack of obvious bleeding point toward a nonorganic problem. Failure to experience vomiting and not being awakened from sleep by discomfort are reassuring factors in your history. It is also important to inform your physician of each and every medicine or pill you are taking, as well as your habits in regard to tobacco, caffeine, and alcohol.

If your physical examination reveals a healthy skin color and normal color in your eye lining (the conjunctiva), anemia resulting from significant blood loss can be excluded. Stable weight is an indication of health as well. With non-ulcer dyspepsia, the abdominal examination usually reveals no abnormality. There is no localized area of tenderness, although the lower end of the breastbone—the cartilaginous end of the sternum called the *xiphoid process*—may be tender when pressed with the fingertips. Most people are unaware of this normal anatomical finding and often are worried when they press on this spot in their self-examination and experience pain. It has absolutely no significance. A normal rectal examination and stool in the rectum that does not contain any hidden or clinical evidence of bleeding are frequent findings in this syndrome that are all to the good.

What Tests Should I Have?

Nowadays no part of the human body is sacred. We can probe every part, insert needles just about everywhere, insert tubes into every orifice, and image every area of the upper intestine and bowel with X-rays (GI series and barium enemas) or sound (abdominal sonogram), scans (gastric emptying tests and the CT scan), as well as magnetic forces (magnetic resonance imaging, or MRI). So it becomes a matter of clinical judgment as to what procedures to put you through to establish the diagnosis and arrive at the most likely alternative diagnoses. It boils down to what else besides non-ulcer dyspepsia we must rule out. Certainly, ulcer disease of the stomach or duodenum is first on our list. Tumors of the stomach are the least likely in the younger patient. Gallbladder disease, especially if there has been an attack or sharp pain, must be taken seriously. Pancreatitis in the male, especially if there has been a history of increasing alcohol intake, should be considered. Possibly gallbladder disease in the female, especially if there is a family history of gallstones, must be ruled out. The irritable bowel syndrome, which can have upper intestinal repercussions and involve gastritis, if your list of medicines includes members of the aspirin family or the nonsteroidal, anti-inflammatory drugs used in arthritis, should not be ignored. Even esophagitis should be considered if there is a question of heartburn or reflux.

Quite a list, you exclaim, and quite expensive too; but the order must depend on the clinical likelihood of each of these entities. The general physical examination has included the rectal stool examination for blood, and of course a routine blood count is indicated to rule out bleeding and anemia. A history of associated and persistent diarrhea should lead to examination of the stools for organisms and parasites. Since your symptoms suggest the upper gastrointestinal tract, imaging of the stomach and upper small bowel (the duodenum) clearly seems the most direct route to follow.

Here the choice lies between the upper GI series, which visualizes the area with barium and X-rays, and upper gastrointestinal endoscopy, which views the interior of these organs and permits color photography, biopsies of tissues, and cultures of the contents of the stomach or duodenum. Your physician's experience—that is, expertise—and estimate of the risks involved play a part in his or her decisions about which route to offer you. I am old-fashioned enough to want a road map provided by X-rays before endoscopy is performed since X-rays are almost totally risk free. However, many experienced colleagues of mine, especially the younger generation of gastroenterologists, prefer to go directly to endoscopy and they may, in the long run, turn out to be right.

If the X-ray provided by the upper GI series does not answer the questions raised by your history and physical examination, then I, too, turn to my well-trained colleagues to perform the upper intestinal endoscopy, which includes the esophagus, stomach, and duodenum. Even though no lesion is seen, I believe biopsies of each organ are in order, to determine whether there is microscopic inflammation. If you have to be put through these procedures, then cultures and smears of the stomach and duodenum to detect *H. pylori*, and especially *Giardia lamblia*, make good sense. The latter organism is rather elusive and may be very difficult to find.

If these studies are not productive, then I would turn to a non-X-ray test—the sonogram—which uses sound waves to image the liver, pancreas, and especially the gallbladder. This is a helpful and risk-free way of eliminating disorders of these organs when supported by functional blood tests of the organs themselves.

When these studies have been complete, we are left very often with a large number of patients with upper intestinal symptoms without obvious cause. To this entity is given the label *non-ulcer dyspepsia* (abbreviated NUD). For some observers, this term is used for symptoms of dyspepsia that elude evaluation and for which apppropriate studies and endoscopy have ruled out organic disease. For other physicians, the condition must exist for more than four weeks for this label to apply.

Now that I Have Been Labeled as Having Non-ulcer Dyspepsia, What Can Be Done About It?

When you learn that the problems of NUD are not easy to treat, you are not surprised because it seems a vague wastebasket that includes a whole gamut of different symptoms, related mainly because they arise high in the gastrointestinal tract. So your doctor will attempt to sort out which symptoms are most disturbing to you and try to fit you into one of several categories in order to give you some relief.

One group of symptoms resembles reflux of acid from the stomach into the esophagus. Others resemble ulcerlike symptoms. Some seem to be related to air swallowing—*aerophagia* is the technical term. Thus it is not surprising to learn that most patients with NUD are treated with antacids and especially histamine II blockers of the Zantac®, Tagamet®, Pepcid®, and Axid® variety. Those who fit into one of these three subgroups seem to respond and do improve.

But a large group of NUD patients appear to have a different kind of difficulty: bloating, a feeling of fullness, flatulence, burping and belching, along with their inability to finish a normal-size meal. They instinctively feel there is something wrong with the emptying of their stomach, so the concept has gradually arisen that some NUD persons are suffering from a motility problem—a problem in the movement of food and fluid through the stomach and duodenum.

NUD Considered as a Motility Problem

The function of the stomach, especially its emptying, needs to be carefully studied in some patients with NUD. Their symptoms seem to be related to the difficulty they experience in emptying their stomach. With scans, it has been learned that liquids leave the stomachs of these patients normally, but there may be a delay in getting the digestive process started and in getting solid food out of the stomach, and so it moves more slowly through the organ. Further studies with pressure-recording devices have shown that this results in part from abnormalities in the pressure of the antrum of the stomach, which is low in these patients. Some sufferers have a disturbance in the control rhythm of the antral muscles. This *dysrhythmia,* which can be analogous to a dysrhythmia of the heart, is probably related to an abnormal pacemaker in the stomach, as in the case of the heart. Unfortunately, at present, we do not have an available "electrocardiogram" for the stomach. Motility disturbances in the upper intestines also seem to be present in some NUD people. Motility scans and antral pressure tracings arouse the suspicion that this condition may be the underlying cause of the individual's discomfort.

DO WE KNOW WHAT CAUSES THESE DISTURBANCES IN MOTILITY?

The straightforward answer is, "We do not."

WHAT ARE THE POSSIBILITIES?

Perhaps when studies are available that can uncover the fine microscopic nature of the upper gut, structural abnormalities of muscles and nerves will be found, as was the case of the curious and disturbing disease of *chronic idiopathic pseudo-obstruction,* which mimics mechanical obstruction anywhere along the gut.

Since women especially suffer from this disorder, hormonal effects may be involved. Local chemical changes in the tissues, not found in blood samples, may also be the culprit. Diabetes certainly can result in failure of the stomach to empty.

I have observed some individuals whose gastric emptying was abruptly slowed after a viral infection, but who recovered spontaneously after weeks or months of distress. Perhaps as in the disease *myasthenia gravis*—in which individuals have difficulty in moving their voluntary muscles—some immunological mechanism alters the ability of the chemical receptors in the stomach and intestinal muscles to respond normally to the presence of a meal in the gut.

Do I Need Other Specialized Tests if I Have Non-ulcer Dyspepsia?

Actually, the only motility test of the upper GI tract that is regularly available in clinical practice is the gastric emptying scan. In this procedure, the patient consumes an isotopically labeled meal of solids and/or liquids, and its exit from the stomach is measured and timed. It is painless and without any significant risk. If your symptoms are present and disturbing, I feel that it is a worthwhile test to undergo even if it may not turn out to be helpful in your individual case. If this emptying scan does reveal problems, it will certainly encourage your doctor to turn to medications that can improve the muscle activity of the stomach and help it empty itself more effectively.

What Drugs Can Help These Motility Disorders?

At present, we have at least three drugs that can stimulate gastrointestinal motility. They are labeled *prokinetic drugs* and include metoclopramide (Reglan®), domperidone (Motilium®), and Cisapride®, with metoclopramide being the longest in use and best known. Domperidone and Cisapride® are widely used throughout the world, but are not yet approved for routine use in the United States. These drugs may be obtained abroad or for compassionate use when an individual enters a clinical study.

Metoclopramide (Reglan®) acts on both the esophageal and stomach muscles and on the brain directly. Its action on the brain makes it a useful drug in curtailing or diminishing nausea, but in some individuals it has the disadvantage of causing involuntary muscle movement or tremors. This calls for prompt cessation of the drug and treatment with antihistamines.

Metoclopramide is particularly valuable because it stimulates esophageal pressure and increases peristalsis, pressure in the lower esophageal sphincter, and contractions of the antral portion of the stomach. The net effect is to move things quickly along the upper GI tract and out of the stomach, thus overcoming some of the symptoms that result from a delay in gastric emptying.

Domperidone (Motilium®) has the advantage of not crossing the blood-brain barrier and not causing any central nervous system side effects. And it controls nausea as well. Like metoclopramide, since it improves stomach emptying by increasing muscle action, it does help some of the symptoms of NUD that have been blamed on the presumed abnormalities of gastric motility.

The third drug of this group, Cisapride®, acts by a different mechanism and avoids the side effects of the other drugs. Indeed, it stimulates the lower bowel and the colon as well; but I have not found this part of its action very effective. While it gains in not having the side effects of Reglan® or Motilium®, its loss is that it has no effect on nausea or vomiting.

More recently it has been discovered that the antibiotic erythromycin also has the ability to empty the stomach. This has been well shown for the delay in gastric motility seen in some individuals with diabetes. Erythromycin is best given intravenously, so it is most useful in an acute situation. When it is given by mouth, the obvious problem is the delay in getting the medication out of the stomach and into the small bowel where it can be absorbed. So we are far from knowing what its exact place should be in our therapy.

Psuedo-Obstruction

In gastroparesis, when the stomach reveals its failure to move its contents along, we look for a mechanical barrier. Sometimes, however, none can be found to explain what looks like and behaves like a mechanical obstruction. In recent years, we have come to realize that in some individuals this false or pseudo-obstruction can affect all parts of the gastrointestinal tract. This syndrome is called *chronic intestinal pseudo-obstruction.*

If it is in the upper gastrointestinal tract, trouble in swallowing, bloating, distention, nausea and vomiting, even pain may be present. In the lower portion of the GI tract, marked abdominal swelling and constipation can occur. Since the contents of the small intestine stagnate, bacteria can proliferate, act on the unabsorbed diet, and cause diarrhea or what we call "bacterial overgrowth."

These sufferers can be young or middle-aged; they may be the only ones in their family to have the trouble, or have brothers and sisters who have the same problem. Often the diagnosis is only given consideration after these individuals have had one or more exploratory operations in the vain hope of relieving the pseudo-obstruction, but nothing grossly abnormal is found.

I am old enough to remember the time when no organic basis could be found or ascribed to account for this condition, but in recent years special staining methods have demonstrated abnormalities in the nerve cells and connections within the walls of the intestine in some sufferers. This is the *neurogenic* form—that is, the form of this disease that has its origin in nerve abnormalities. In other forms, electronmicroscopy and special strains reveal abnormalities of the smooth muscle; this is the *myopathic* form.

How Is the Diagnosis Confirmed?

Manometric pressure tracings of the esophagus, discussed in Chapter 3 in the section on "Functional Tests," will reveal some abnormalities. One hesitates to make the diagnosis of chronic intestinal pseudo-obstruction in their absence. They are usually present, even if a particular individual does not have problems swallowing.

Pressure studies measured by an electrical recording system of the upper small bowel and rectosigmoid section of the colon (lowest section of the large bowel) in the fasting state and after eating can also help pinpoint the diagnosis. Most biopsies taken during endoscopic procedures either do not go deep enough into the cell layer or have not been studied adequately by special stains or electronmicroscopy to help make the diagnosis. One really needs a biopsy of the entire thickness of the wall, something we are not likely to do except during surgery.

What Can Be Done to Help Individuals with This Rather Rare Condition?

First, we can try to avoid unnecessary exploratory surgery of the abdomen. Malnutrition can be completely overcome by *total parenteral nutrition* (TPN), a procedure in which the person is fed intravenously for long periods of time. Bacterial overgrowth can be well handled by antibiotics. The full effects of our newer prokinetic agents have not yet been worked out, but occasionally marked improvement has been reported. Finally, we can make sure that intestinal infections are handled promptly, because these can create problems more severe than the original complaint. Disturbances in the amounts of electrolytes in the blood—such as a low potassium or chloride concentration—can make the obstruction worse and are easily corrected. In addition, we should be careful to avoid, if we can, many of the neurally active drugs, especially the tricyclical antidepressants, which slow the intestine down. Unfortunately, some of these individuals have Parkinson's disease and need these drugs for the management of this condition.

Labeled or nonlabeled, non-ulcer dyspepsia makes many individuals very uncomfortable. Their distress is no less real because we can find no organic basis for it at present. Nor is it enough for physicians to glibly pass it off as being "stress related."

Like the irritable bowel syndrome, since the diagnosis of non-ulcer dyspepsia is a diagnosis of exclusion, I cannot see any way that those who have these disturbing symptoms and sensations can skip the needed diagnostic studies that this chapter has outlined. If I had these complaints, I would want as positive a diagnosis of my condition as my physician could give me.

Often, many individuals are relieved both mentally and physically by the assurance of the nonorganic nature of their complaints, while many others desire and want relief and help. If your NUD fits the acid reflux pattern in the esophagus or resembles ulcerlike symptoms, then you should be treated as if you had these disorders to prevent their possible development. If your symptoms and studies point toward a disturbance in the motility process which moves the contents of the stomach along in a smooth coordinated pattern, then a trial of the prokinetic agents is worth making, after being alerted to the possible side effects of some of the current medications. When these medications work, the result is very gratifying indeed.

7

All Chest Pain
Is Not Heart Pain

Throughout this book, I deal with upper intestinal digestive complaints that range from the mildest to the most severe in intensity. Yet none is so frightening as an episode of severe anterior—that is, front—chest pain, which makes the average individual fear he or she is having a heart attack.

True *angina*—that is, pain arising from the heart because of difficulties in the flow of blood through the coronary arteries—usually can be distinguished from chest pain, which arises from the esophagus. The esophageal pain has nothing to do with effort or walking or climbing stairs; it can occur at night while a person is at rest or even awaken the person from sleep. Individuals who have problems in swallowing can also experience this intense pain. Sometimes the swallowing problems are quite troublesome to the sufferer, and yet others may feel only minor discomfort. Some persons complain of heartburn, but the heartburn does not disturb them too much. It is the tight feeling behind the breastbone which is so threatening.

Because the chest pain coming from the esophagus can mimic the anginal pain of heart disease, most patients and their physicians consider the heart first. When the cardiovascular system had been exonerated, then attention focuses on the esophagus. Doctors are now well aware of this condition and may consider the esophagus earlier in the diagnostic considerations than they did in years past. Almost everyone who turns up in my office with these symptoms has already had an electrocardiogram. Some have had various cardiac stress tests, and a few, especially older patients, may even have had catheterization of the coronary arteries and dye flow studies performed with angiographic pictures of the heart arteries.

The common esophageal causes of the chest pain that may imitate the angina of heart disease are (1) gastroesophageal reflux of acid into the esophagus; (2) disturbances in the motility function of the esophagus—that is, the ability of the esophagus to move things along; and (3) the irritable esophageal syndrome. Let us consider each of these in turn.

1. *Gastroesophageal reflux,* which we looked at in detail in Chapter 4, which considered heartburn, esophagitis, and hiatal hernia, may give rise to pain that the patient distinguishes from his ordinary heartburn, especially by its intense "burning."
2. The *motility abnormalities* include several types:
   a. The condition of *achalasia* (also known as cardiospasm), which has nothing to do with the heart, results from the failure of the lower sphincter of the esophagus to relax along with the swallowing reflex. The pain may be very severe, have little relation to meals, and may awaken the patient from sleep. We discuss this syndrome in the Appendix (in the section "Difficulties in Swallowing").
   b. Another variant of achalasia—*vigorous achalasia*—has one feature in addition to those present in ordinary achalasia: the act of swallowing leads to bursts of repeated esophageal contractions that do not move food

along or forward. This causes pain and difficulty in getting food down.

c. *Diffuse esophageal spasm* (DES) is a spastic condition of the esophagus in which swallowing gives rise to a series of many, long, high-pressure waves that do not travel anywhere and do not move anything along.

3. And, finally, in addition to gastroesophageal reflux and the motility disturbances, we must consider (which we do in a moment) the *irritable esophageal syndrome* in which the esophagus is supersensitive to acid reflux and to motor disturbances.

Irritable Esophageal Syndrome (IES)

We all know about the irritable bowel syndrome (IBS). So many have it, including a great many who have never even visited a physician to confirm its existence. The combination of lower abdominal pain or discomfort, distention, and disturbances in bowel movement—diarrhea or constipation, or an alternation between these two extremes of bowel movements—make up the classic textbook description. The diagnosis at present is one of exclusion, arrived at only after your doctor has ruled out organic disease of the colon by appropriate blood and stool examinations, sigmoidoscopy, X-rays, and/or colonoscopy. The causes of irritable bowel syndrome are still obscure. But the opinion is growing that it is a disorder of the contractions of the smooth muscle of the colon influenced by a number of factors that may include mechanical distention or stretching, food residues and their chemical constituents, the release of intestinal hormones (chemical messengers which send signals from one area of the gastrointestinal tract to another), as well as psychological and physical stress. The result of these elements produces dysrhythmia of the bowel, similar to a disturbance of the heart rhythm (arrhythmia).

The reason for this digression on irritable bowel syndrome is that we are gradually realizing that these disturbances occur not only in the colon, but in the entire bowel, including the small intestine. Of course, the stomach has long been the subject of studies of the effects of emotional stress on its workings, but no area in the gastrointestinal tract is exempt from those disturbances of muscle contraction. The concept of irritable bowel syndrome has now been extended to the esophagus. *The irritable esophagus is often a part of the irritable gut.*

How Does the Irritable Esophagus Show Itself?

Pain and discomfort, a sense of tightness behind the breastbone not related to effort or exertion (unlike heart disease), rarely difficulty in swallowing—these are the chief complaints of irritable esophagus. Often just the sense that there is something there as you struggle to describe it and you point to your breastbone. It feels different from heartburn with its characteristic burning sensation; yet sometimes you feel it is difficult to distinguish it from heartburn.

X-rays of the esophagus or a view into its interior with endoscopy reveal no gross abnormalities and often biopsies do not reveal even minimal inflammation. Very often, before the esophagus is turned to as a possible site of the trouble, you have had a careful cardiac evaluation, including resting electrocardiograms and a variety of cardiac stress tests during exercise which have eliminated the heart as the cause of your discomfort.

At this point, tests directed to the functioning of the esophagus and the pressure waves that move the contents along may be the only way of pinpointing the problem. Measurements of the pressure and the movement of pressure waves by *esophageal manometry* (see Chapter 3, "Functional Tests") can verify that periods of increased high-pressure waves coincide with your distress. The pain may also occur at times when these waves fail to move forward in an orderly fashion. Even if manometry fails to show high-pressure waves as disorganized or uncoordinated waves of contraction, your distress may arise for another reason.

Your threshold for experiencing discomfort in the esophagus

may be low and thus you may be very sensitive to any changes in pressure. Just as in irritable bowel syndrome, patients feel full of gas and yet their bowels contain only normal amounts of air. They are uncomfortable because their threshold for feeling pain or distention is very low. So in the irritable esophagus, your threshold for pain—that is, the level at which you perceive discomfort—is lower than your neighbor's. This can be discovered through a simple procedure in which a little balloon filled with air is placed in the esophagus and blown up. If this test reproduces your discomfort at very low pressures we have proof of an irritable esophagus. Another test uses very dilute acid, which may also reproduce pain in the sensitive esophagus.

At this point, as in IBS, we must consider the possible role emotion or other stresses may play in the IES (irritable esophageal syndrome). In the laboratory, researchers have showed that abnormal esophageal contractions and discomfort can be induced in healthy individuals using unpredictable noises or unpleasant interviews. In some patients with IES, these unpredictable noises or difficult intellectual tasks initiated significant and painful increases in pressure in the esophagus. Now that it is possible to monitor patients during real-life situations, we can observe and record esophageal pressure during various activities for periods as long as 24 hours (similar to the Holter monitor used in cardiac arrhythmias). We can then attempt to relate these physiological fluctuations to the individual's moods and feelings. Just how emotional factors affect the muscular activity of the esophagus, by what neural or chemical messages, is not known at present; but the fact of their reality has become clearer as work in this field continues to advance.

What Can Be Done About the Irritable Esophageal Syndrome

Just as in the irritable bowel, I believe the obvious irritants we take in—caffeine, alcohol, nicotine—should be eliminated. The more elusive irritants of daily life are harder to track down; they are possibly more important than the single dramatic shocks of tragic life situations. Sometimes the newer calcium channel blockers can give relief. Taken on a regular basis, they help to dampen the esophageal responses. It goes almost without saying that all attempts to reduce psychic stress are worthwhile. In addition, it has been recorded that some medicines which reduce pain perception are helpful.

How Do We Prove that Some Chest Pain Is Due to the Esophagus?

To distinguish these different causes, we need to record the pressure curves in the esophagus and the response to swallowing, and determine whether acidic gastric contents get back into the esophagus. In some research centers it is possible to monitor what happens to pressure and acidity over 24-hour periods with minimal discomfort and to find out whether your pain is associated with reflux or motor abnormalities, or both.

In addition to these monitoring tests, there are three provocative tests that will help at times. All three tests attempt to reproduce your pain, one by dripping diluted acid into the esophagus (the Bernstein test), another by giving a drug (edrophonium, Tensilon®) which may stimulate the muscle of the esophagus and thus may reproduce your discomfort in a momentary attack, the third by distending the esophagus with a balloon to bring on discomfort.

HOW OFTEN IS THE ESOPHAGUS THE CAUSE OF CHEST PAIN AND WHICH SPECIAL TESTS DO I NEED TO BE SURE IT IS NOT ANGINA?

In one carefully conducted study of a series, 60 patients whose heart had been cleared by the most sophisticated techniques were studied to determine the nature of their pain. Half were shown to be suffering from esophageal pain. This is an important point to keep in mind if your doctor suggests that you undergo monitoring and some tests.

What did this group of 30 patients have? Forty percent had gastroesophageal reflux, 40 percent fell into the irritable esophageal syndrome, and 20 percent had problems with motility (moving food along).

What Is the Therapeutic Gain of All This Testing?

Obviously to be assured that you do not have any life-threatening heart disease is the first and most important gain. Knowing the nature of your pain will also allow your physician to recommend a course of treatment to eliminate your discomfort. Gastroesophageal reflux can be treated quite successfully by our current medical programs, as outlined in Chapter 4; in rare instances, it may be "cured" by operation. The motor disorders, such as achalasia, respond to medications containing nitrates or the calcium channel blockers, endoscopic dilatation, or the operation which cuts the lower esophageal sphincter—the Heller cardiomyotomy. The medical approach to irritable esophagus is more difficult, but this condition can be managed by a judicious diet, an improvement in eating habits, medications that alleviate pain, plus better handling of stress.

A Pause for a Newer Concept

Now that I have reassured you that we can, without too much difficulty, separate the innocent chest pain arising from the esophagus from the threatening pain of coronary artery disease, I have to throw you a curve.

We need to consider a recent idea that suggests that a few individuals may have quite normal results from electrocardiograms, cardiac stress tests, and even angiograms, and may still be suffering from *microvascular angina*. This term refers to pain that arises from the heart during transient, minor episodes when blood flow through the smallest vessels (not abnormal on the angiogram) to the heart muscle is not enough to meet the heart's requirement.

The good news is that individuals with microvascular angina have a good long-term prognosis and respond well to calcium channel-blocking drugs that relax the smooth muscle and dilate the blood vessels it contains.

To make an absolute diagnosis of this condition would require arduous and expensive testing using an angiogram and intravenous drugs. Perhaps less invasive tests will soon be forthcoming, but, in the meantime, I would be most reluctant to subject my patients to this form of testing. I am content to be reassured and, in turn, to reassure my patients that if their electrocardiogram, stress testing, and angiogram are negative, their hearts are healthy. Especially if the esophageal manometry reveals abnormality in motor function, an individual's prognosis is good and effective treatment can be planned.

Since our treatment of reflux and other esophageal pain is successful, I would suggest a vigorous trial of all antireflux methods and acid-blocking techniques before proceeding to tests for microvascular angina.

8

The Gallbladder in the Stone Age

The gallbladder nestles in the upper portion of the abdomen, on the right side, just beneath the liver and under the right ribs. As you will recall from the overview of the workings of the upper digestive tract in Chapter 1, the gallbladder is the receptacle for the temporary storage of bile which it receives continuously from the liver, but which it needs to discharge into the intestine only from time to time for the digestion of fats in the course of a meal (*Figure 7*).

The main problem associated with the gallbladder when things go wrong is that it makes stones, which can cause serious difficulties and pain. The point of my title for this chapter is that current emphasis is fixed on the problem of gallstones. Future horizons will probably be wider and will focus on prevention.

A second problem, which I think is equally important, is that the gallbladder is blamed unfairly for any discomfort in this area, for any indigestion remotely connected with fatty foods. In this chapter, I hope to sort out for you the real, from the alleged, problems of the gallbladder.

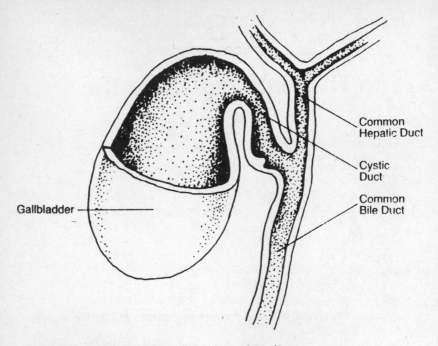

FIGURE 7. Diagram of the gallbladder and its ducts.

Gallbladder Disease

The gallbladder gets blamed for digestive problems so often because gallstone disease is so common. Somewhere between 10 and 20 percent of the world's population have gallstones. It has also been estimated that the majority of adults above the age of 60 years have gallstones.

Who Gets Gallstones?

Some families have the tendency to form gallstones, so there is a genetic factor. The Pima Indians in the Southwestern United States, for example, have a high incidence of gallstones, perhaps 85 to 90 percent of the women and 70 to 80 percent of the men are affected. Women are prone to gallstone formation and this susceptibility increases with pregnancy. Men also have their share, although far smaller than that of women.

The overweight suffer more, especially those individuals who are obese and attempt to drop pounds by trying crash weight-reduction programs. While you might suppose that individuals with elevated levels of cholesterol in their blood are more likely to have gallstones, this is not the case; but some people with increased blood fats—triglycerides—do have a greater chance of forming stones. Some drugs, like older forms of the contraceptive pill, seem to have played a role in inducing cholesterol stones among the women who used them. While the young can have stones, the incidence of gallstones increases with age, especially as we approach middle age.

What Kinds of Stones Are There?

All gallstones are not the same. The more important ones, because they are the most frequent, are the cholesterol stones, which account for 70 percent of the gallstones of patients in Europe and the United States. These cholesterol stones contain more than 70 percent cholesterol. Some are pure cholesterol and form only one stone; others are called *mixed cholesterol stones*. These mixed stones—usually more than one—contain calcium as well as a mucus protein center.

The other type of gallstone is the pigment stone, which is either brown or black in color. The brown ones are soft and break up easily; the black ones are hard and brittle. Both contain calcium along with the breakdown products of hemoglobin, bilirubin, as well as a mucus protein portion at their core.

What Causes Gallstones?

Let us look at pigment stones first because they are less frequent and less important. They are formed when the bile contains excessive amounts of bilirubin—the breakdown product of hemoglobin, which is contained in our red blood cells. Bilirubin will settle out of solution—"precipitate," as we say—very easily. In contrast to cholesterol stones, we know little about what sets this process in motion, but we do know that these stones occur in people with cirrhosis of the liver. Individuals whose red blood cells are destroyed more rapidly than normal will also form this type of stone; this group would include people with chronic hemolytic anemia, sickle cell disease, and malaria. Suture material—thread left in from previous surgery—may be instrumental in bringing down pigment stones in the bile ducts.

You should remember, however, that for any gallstones to form one needs a gallbladder. Stones found in the bile ducts after gallbladder surgery are either left over from a prior operation or form in a leftover portion of the gallbladder that has somehow not been removed completely. Stones formed in the common bile duct in individuals who have had no operations are almost invariably stones that have moved from the gallbladder into the duct passage system.

Unlike pigment stones, cholesterol stones result from the secretion of an abnormal bile by the liver. The trouble with this bile is that it is supersaturated—that is, oversaturated—with cholesterol. Ordinarily, bile is able to dissolve the cholesterol it transports out of the liver because of its unique chemical composition. The most important dissolving components of bile are the bile acids made by the liver from cholesterol. At present, we believe the supersaturated bile results from an imbalance between the overproduction of cholesterol by the liver and its simultaneous and concomitant underproduction of bile acids. But many of us have cholesterol-saturated bile from time to time without the cholesterol crystallizing and joining together to form stones, especially when we are fasting. So something else must be wrong as well. One needs to have trouble in the gallbladder, for it is there that these cholesterol crystals settle out.

In the gallbladder several factors are at work. First, irregular meal patterns may lead to a longer storage time for bile in the gallbladder in human beings than in other mammals. Second, there appears to be a substance in the gallbladder bile that hastens the process of nucleation—that is, that gets the process going. Third, the gallbladder may not empty itself effectively in association with cholesterol stones. Fourth, inflammation of the gallbladder wall may interfere with that organ's ability to absorb cholesterol and thus reduce the supersaturation. Finally, gallstones may stimulate mucus which further traps cholesterol crystals. So in the end both a supersaturated bile, made by the liver, and disorders of the gallbladder are implicated when we form cholesterol crystals and then stones.

The imbalance between production of cholesterol in the liver and inadequate secretion of bile salts helps us to understand something of great interest to individuals with inflammatory bowel disease, especially Crohn's disease. We have known for a long time that they suffer from more gallbladder disease than might be expected to happen by chance. The reason is quite simple: they suffer from a lack of bile because they fail to recapture these bile acids in the intestine; this occurs because of disease in the ileum or because they have lost their ileum due to surgery.

How Do Gallstones Show Themselves?

Gallstones may never show themselves, even if you have had them for some time. These are the *silent stones,* which often are discovered by accident. An X-ray of the abdomen, done for some other reason, may show these cholesterol stones when they contain calcium and cast a shadow on the X-ray film. Or more frequently nowadays, a sonogram of the abdomen, looking for trouble elsewhere, may disclose the characteristic picture of cholesterol stones, which need not contain calcium.

In contrast to these silent stones, others may speak up very loudly. These are the ones we are really concerned about. They cause trouble in several different ways. Often they attempt to get out of the gallbladder when it contracts to empty itself; this causes severe pain. There are few pains as bad as this: having a kidney stone, or attempting to pass one, and having a baby through the birth canal are more severe; but few other abdominal disorders cause pain with the intensity of gallstones. Typically, the pain is in the area of the gallbladder—the right upper portion of the abdomen. Often it spreads across the right side of the abdomen to the right flank and right side of the back, occasionally to the left side of the abdomen. Characteristically, the pain may spread to the right shoulder blade and even to the right shoulder. This pain may cause nausea and vomiting, but not regularly.

Along with the pain comes tenderness on examination by just touching the area. The gallbladder may become inflamed, causing chills and fever. A stone may become jammed in the neck of the gallbladder, blocking the exit of bile and making the organ swollen and tense. This causes a chemical inflammation of the gallbladder, known as *acute cholecystitis.* Or a stone or stones may get out of the gallbladder and into the bile ducts, blocking the flow of bile into the intestine. The bile will then back up into the blood, and the patient becomes jaundiced. This condition is caused by the yellow color of the pigment in the bile (bilirubin). Often the whites of the eye are the earliest place where jaundice can be detected in a good light. Later, as the amount of bile in the blood increases, the yellow colors all the skin, even the lining of the mouth, and becomes quite obvious. Finally, the bile spills over into the kidney, and the urine becomes dark—often as dark as strong tea or cola. Along with the yellow pigment of the bile that enters the bloodstream, bile acids from the liver make their way as well. These acids cause itching all over the body when they are deposited in the skin.

Typically an attack of this kind, with the accompanying pain—*biliary colic,* as physicians label it—occurs shortly after a rich meal with fatty foods and cream; but not necessarily so. Moreover, the pain may not be horrendous; it may be quite mild and nagging in character.

I have just described the classic symptoms of a gallstone attack, but the pain may also spread across the front part of the chest, and the first thought the patient may have is "My God, I am having a heart attack!" So this possibility must be ruled out.

One further point needs to be mentioned here. The pain may spread across the upper abdomen to the left side and be quite strong, feeling as though it is boring through to the left side of the back. The patient now feels better sitting up, rather than lying down, or even better leaning forward. The added pain in this new location results from the spread of inflammation into the adjacent *pancreas*—a point we will talk about at greater length in Chapter 9 on the pancreas and pancreatitis.

Should One Get Rid of All Gallstones?

Even before we discuss how to treat gallstones, the first question to be answered is: "Do all persons with gallstones need treatment?" For stones to be discovered is no reason to assume they must now be treated in some way. The silent, accidentally discovered ones may not necessarily need to be removed or dissolved. Of course, we would all be better off if we had no stones and no worry of their possible threat in the future; but I see no need to do something just because the stones are there. Even the very rare possibility that a tumor might arise in a gallbladder filled with stones at some remote time in the future is no reason, in my opinion, to routinely remove all gallstones. Not merely the cost, but the risks of this form of treatment are not justified by such a wholesale attack as would be required for this common condition.

We once thought that persons with diabetes should routinely have their gallbladders removed if they contained stones. The mistaken belief was that these individuals would have a greater likelihood of getting ill in the future as a result of the stones and that they would have a more severe course of the disease than otherwise healthy individuals. Modern well-controlled studies have shown that these beliefs have no real basis in fact.

On the other hand, if a young woman of childbearing age is discovered to have a gallbladder filled with small stones that might complicate her pregnancy, I would certainly consider having her take care of this problem before she becomes pregnant. Small stones can more easily get out of the gallbladder and block the flow of bile in the ducts, in contrast to one large stone.

So much for the silent stones. What about those that have announced themselves? I mean those that have caused an attack of biliary colic, the severe pain I have described. I do not advise an automatic reprisal just because you have had an episode. I would take into account the circumstances of the attack and what possibly may have triggered it. If someone has had but one attack, the decision whether to wait for a second one before doing something is a joint patient–doctor decision. The young woman of childbearing age I mentioned above would be wise to avoid trouble in the future. However, if your first and only attack of biliary colic was complicated by jaundice, chills, and fever, blood tests that reveal an abnormal liver, acute inflammation of the gallbladder or pancreatitis, my vote is to treat the disease vigorously.

What Kind of Treatment Can We Now Choose?

Up until recently we had only one method of getting rid of gallstones—removing the gallbladder. Although we know that the liver makes bad bile—bile supersaturated with cholesterol—stones form only in the gallbladder. If we want to take care of the gallstones, we must remove the gallbladder. Simply removing the stones does no good; the abnormal bile would re-form stones in the gallbladder still in place. This lesson has been well learned over the past century.

But removing the gallbladder (*cholecystectomy*) means a major abdominal operation and its attendant risks. Yet done correctly it solves the problem of gallstones once and for all.

What Are the Pros and Cons of This Operation?

I have already stated: "no gallbladder, no stones." This certainly holds true of cholesterol stones, the prevalent variety. The gallbladder is a dispensable organ; the rat, the horse, and the pigeon have no gallbladder. Hence, Hamlet's well-known quotation: "I am pigeon-livered, I do lack gall." By and large, you can live perfectly well and digest your meals adequately without a gallbladder. Since the gallbladder's main function is to store bile, its removal leads to the flow of bile more or less continuously into the duodenum. For a few individuals, the continuous entry of bile into the intestine may act as a mild cathartic or laxative, while for some, this actually corrects mild constipation. On the other hand, the continuous presence of bile in the upper intestine may lead to irritation of the stomach (*bile gastritis*) if individuals have any condition which leads to regurgitation of bile into the stomach, such as a previous ulcer operation, or regurgitation into the esophagus (*bile esophagitis*), if they have any condition, such as a hiatal hernia, which would favor this regurgitation, or if they experience a delay in gastric emptying. But for the majority of individuals, removal of the gallbladder solves the problem at once.

What About the Down Side? What Are the Risks and Problems?

First, there are, of course, the general risks of anesthesia and abdominal surgery, the severity of which depends on your age, general health, and the presence or absence of heart, lung, or kidney disease. If your doctor, after careful examination and evaluation, decides you are fit to be operated on, the risks are those a prudent person would accept. The operation for gallbladder removal in a modern hospital, with good anesthesia and competent surgical and medical attendants, is the most satisfactory cure for this condition, even in our era of rising medical costs. In fact, this operation may be the most economical way to handle the problem, especially for those with a long lifetime ahead of them.

What can go wrong as a result of this attempt to remove the gallbladder surgically? First, stones may be left over. Some may have entered the bile ducts to begin with or inadvertently tipped over into the duct during the operation. While this, on occasion, may occur, the chances are very slight nowadays, since most surgeons use radiological or endoscopic methods to be sure no stone is left behind. They can accomplish this without having to open the common bile duct surgically and without risking injury to that delicate narrow tube. If a stone or stones should be left over, there are a number of techniques for retrieving them in the postoperative period.

Injury to the common bile duct is the most serious surgical mishap that can occur during the surgeon's attempt to remove the entire gallbladder and its short cystic duct (see *Figure 7*). Injuries may cause bile to leak from a hole in the common bile duct, and scarring of any part of the duct may lead to obstruction of the duct, which will interfere with the flow of bile and result in pain. Fortunately, this kind of major injury to the common bile duct is quite rare, but ducts have been damaged quite inadvertently. However, the meticulous care surgeons exercise to avoid injuring the duct may also lead them to stay as far away from the common bile duct as possible and so leave a part of the cystic duct behind or, even rarer, a part of the gallbladder itself. The network of plumbing left behind—the *cystic duct stump,* as it is called—may actually become a mini-gallbladder and form stones or contain some undiscovered ones. Yet, on balance, when one considers the vast number of gallbladder operations done each year, cholecystectomy is one of the safest and most satisfactory abdominal operations performed these days.

When I started to draft this section a short time ago, I would have concluded at this point; but since then a new twist has been added to gallbladder surgery. It is now possible to remove the gallbladder without opening up the abdominal wall in a formal operation. The procedure is called *laparoscopic cholecystectomy*.

Laparoscopic Cholecystectomy

Without making a formal incision, a surgeon can now look into the abdominal peritoneal cavity by inserting an instrument, the *laparoscope,* into that cavity through a small opening in the belly wall. After filling the abdomen with gas, in this case carbon dioxide, the surgeon is able to look around and often visualize many intra-abdominal organs. This technique has been used most frequently and routinely to see the pelvic organs in women and to tie off their fallopian tubes as a contraceptive device. In recent years, surgeons have been able to grasp the appendix and remove it through the same small opening in the abdominal wall. Recently refined by

French physicians, the laparoscopic approach can also enable the surgeon to remove the gallbladder rather quickly. This shortens operating time, reduces the patient's postoperative discomfort remarkably, and cuts the hospital stay to one to two days. It, too, like the more formal operation, requires general anesthesia.

Unfortunately, this method does not allow the surgeon to explore the common bile duct to see if there are any stones left there; so there must be thorough imaging and laboratory studies to indicate that there is no obstruction to the flow of bile in the common bile duct. In the short time that surgeons skilled in this technique have been able to do this operation, I have already seen patients in whom stones of the common duct were left behind or tipped over inadvertently into the common bile duct. So, at the moment, although my stance is guarded and I am waiting to accumulate more information and experience beore arriving at a definitive opinion regarding this operation, which is bound to become very popular, my early experience leads me to believe that, *with proper selection,* this technique will prove a most useful contribution to the gallstone problem. My continuing experience leads me to believe that laparoscopic cholecystectomy will become a permanent option open to my patients.

What About the Newer Methods of Dissolving or Crushing Gallstones?

Laparoscopic surgery is still surgery and so we all have long been looking forward to ways of dissolving gallstones through medication and, more recently, hoping to crush them as the urologists have been crushing kidney stones for some time now. There are two major modern methods for dissolving gallstones in the gallbladder. The best studied method that has been tried more often than any other is the *oral bile salt therapy*—medication taken by mouth that alters the composition of bile. A second method—more experimental and in use for a much shorter period—is *contact dissolution* of gallstones: that is, the use of chemicals that are put directly into the gallbladder to dissolve the stone or stones.

ORAL BILE SALT TREATMENT

When we are looking at the possibility of dissolving gallstones by taking pills by mouth, we are talking about cholesterol stones only. Pigment stones cannot be dissolved and stones containing calcium are resistant to dissolution.

This new procedure was introduced about 15 years ago when Alan Hoffman and his associates at the Mayo Clinic discovered that feeding patients the bile salt chenodeoxycholic acid (CDCA), a normal bile acid, solubolized the cholesterol in the bile; continued feeding led to dissolution of the gallstones. This brilliant observation opened up a whole array of drug treatments in the modern era.

For this method to work, the stone must be composed of cholesterol. And while a gallbladder with many stones can be treated, the stones have to be small—no larger than 1.5 centimeters. (Remember that 1 inch equals 2.2 centimeters.) For this drug treatment to be attempted, your gallbladder must be functioning; that is, it must be viewed on X-ray after you take an oral dye. The X-ray picture will reveal the bile as it passes into and out of the gallbladder.

A low cholesterol diet and one dose of CDCA at bedtime are prescribed; obese individuals require larger doses. Undesirable side effects include diarrhea and modest reversible changes in certain liver function tests, which are monitored throughout treatment. Unfortunately, the method takes time since small stones may take up to six months to dissolve. Large stones may require as much as two years of continuous therapy. And yet, in spite of progress, complete disappearance of stones occurs in perhaps no more than 25 percent of subjects.

Another bile salt, ursodeoxycholic acid (UDCA), which has been sold over the counter in Japan for 20 years or more to help in the treatment of biliary distress, is free of the considerable side effects of CDCA and works at lower dosage levels. UDCA dissolves stones somewhat differently from CDCA, and investigators have been trying combination therapies with both bile acids with some success.

In addition to the side effects already mentioned and the slowness of the entire treatment program, there is another important drawback to this approach. Since the gallbladder is still in place, there is a tendency for the stones to recur after being dissolved. It is said about one-third of the stones will be re-formed within three years; by seven years in half the patients. So full dosage treatment must be continued indefinitely with this as yet expensive drug program. Low-dose bile acid treatment with UDCA used continuously does not seem to do the trick.

From this account, you can see that the use of bile acids by mouth must have a very limited place in the treatment of stones at present, even with the modified side effects of UDCA. However, in those with recurrent colic who are too sick because of other diseases of the heart, lung, or kidneys, this method does offer a reasonable approach that can be used in the short term as a tolerable alternative to gallbladder surgery.

A WORD ABOUT CONTACT DISSOLUTION OF GALLSTONES

A more experimental method of dissolving stones in the gallbladder, also developed at the Mayo Clinic, consists of injecting a chemical substance—methy terbutyl ether (MTBE)—directly into the gallbladder by a catheter passed through the abdominal wall and through the liver. MTBE is foul smelling and can cause a burning pain in the upper abdomen. A person may also experience nausea and vomiting, even damage to the kidneys, if the MTBE escapes from the gallbladder. The procedure may take five- to seven-hour cycles in which the medication is instilled and withdrawn from the gallbladder. These cycles may have to be repeated at a subsequent session.

From this brief description, you can see that it is a method which requires the expertise of its inventors for the time being, and much more reported experience before I would advocate it to patients with a functioning gallbladder and cholesterol stones.

WHAT ABOUT CRUSHING GALLBLADDER STONES?

This method, called *extracorporeal shock-wave lithotripsy* (ESWL), is an expensive, noninvasive, and, in my opinion, still experimental way of splitting gallstones into a powder. The early machines that generated a shock wave required the patient to be submerged in a water bath and anesthetized or heavily sedated. The new lithotriptors (stone crushers) have the patient lie in a waterbed for one to two hours, and no sedation is required. Like other nonsurgical methods that I have been writing about, the patient must have a functioning gallbladder and cholesterol stones, not pigment stones. The stones must be small, and the gallbladder must not contain more than three, which cannot be calcified. In addition, in the reported studies from Germany, the patients received CDCA and UDCA—bile salts—by mouth for 12 days before treatment, and they continued these medications for at least three months after the complete disappearance of the stones. Almost all of the stones were shattered and cleared out of the gallbladder after 18 months of bile salt therapy, but about one-third of patients had an attack of biliary pain of the colicky variety and some bleeding into the kidney. Most regrettable is the fact that at present only patients with three small stones are suitable for the technique—probably less than 10 percent of all gallstone patients. All groups have had their best results when the method was used in combination with UDCA by mouth for considerable periods of time following the crushing procedure.

This technique may be improved in the future to handle calcium-containing stones and those patients with more than three stones; but I prefer to wait before recommending this experimental procedure to my patients.

Summing Up the Options

From this discussion, you can easily deduce that pending further improvements in shock wave treatment I prefer surgical removal of the gallbladder for stones for those who really need it, anticipating that laparoscopic removal of the gallbladder will be a most useful addition to the surgical choices. I am reserving chemical dissolution for those few patients whose medical conditions do not allow them to undergo an operation.

Two Hard Questions Regarding the Gallbladder

So far we have been considering what to do about your gallstones because you really need to do something. They have been giving you trouble, mainly pain, which fits the pattern of colic.

Now we face two hard questions: First, your pain sounds and feels like biliary colic, but tests do not show the stones. What could be done in such a case? Second, tests have revealed gallstones, but are they the cause of your distress?

How Can We Prove that the Gallbladder Is the Cause of Your Pain? Your Discomfort Has All the Earmarks of Biliary Colic, and Yet All the Current Tests Do Not Help. What Can We Do Next?

At present, when a patient has the typical severe upper right quadrant pain so characteristic of biliary colic, whether or not they are jaundiced, we rely on the abdominal sonogram to prove that the stones are the cause. This test is highly reliable and gives additional information on whether the stones are blocking the ducts.

But what to do if the sonogram does not prove the point? We can rely on the standard test of many years ago—the oral cholecystogram (OCG). In this procedure, an X-ray is done after the subject has taken a dye by mouth, which passes through the liver and is concentrated in the gallbladder. This test may reveal multiple stones, which appear as a line on the X-ray. Sometimes, however, the gallbladder may not show up on the X-ray, even after a double dose of dye. This is strong evidence that the gallbladder is diseased and probably contains stones.

If both sonogram and cholecystogram are negative, we must consider the possibility that the colic is not being caused by visible, large stones, called *macroliths,* but instead by tiny crystals of cholesterol, called *microliths*. To test for these tiny stones, we can try a much older test and look for the presence of these cholesterol crystals in the bile, which we used to do routinely before the modern imaging era. For this procedure, a sample of bile is obtained from the duodenum with a very small tube that the patient swallows. A synthetic form of the hormone *cholecystokinin* is administered to stimulate the gallbladder to contract and empty its bile. Through the use of a special microscope which uses polarized light, the bile is carefully examined and a search for cholesterol crystals is made, both immediately and after some days of storage under controlled conditions. If cholesterol crystals are detected, your physician has very reliable evidence that your gallbladder contains cholesterol stones.

Sometimes all these tests fail to give us the information we sorely need to prove the existence of biliary tract disease. An avenue I've sometimes used to help in solving this puzzle is to ask the subject to obtain blood tests at the height of an attack. The purpose here is to prove that there is some temporary, and often slight, obstruction to the flow of bile that can be measured in the bilirubin of the blood. So I give my patients a note to carry around with them, and urge them to go to the nearest doctor or emergency room to have blood drawn to detect specific substances in the blood. If a bad attack occurs in the middle of the night, the test need not be run as an emergency, since the blood can be put in cold storage and tests performed by regular laboratory staff the next morning. On occasion, this has been very helpful in establishing the diagnosis. Even so, at times, with only frustrating negative results, we must simply wait until there is clear evidence that the gallbladder is at fault. Sometimes the dramatic appearance of jaundice and its yellowing of the skin and eyeballs in the midst of an episode of colic clinches the case. Now for the really hard question.

Are Your Gallstones the Cause of Your Distress?

We routinely associate upper right quadrant abdominal pain of varying degrees with the gallbladder. We blame the gallbladder for our intolerance of fatty foods and for our belching or burping. Since gallstones are so common, as I have already pointed out, the gallbladder becomes the suspected culprit and surgery is often suggested.

But unless the gallbladder is the cause of distress, removing *that* organ is a futile treatment. The patient will continue to have this distress—labeled *postcholecystectomy syndrome*—and a frustrating search begins to determine what went wrong during the operation. The only thing that went wrong in most cases was the decision to remove the gallbladder. Occasionally, the unneeded surgery may have injured the bile ducts, but this rarely causes biliary tract disease.

Much careful clinical study has shown that the mere presence of small discomfort in the upper right abdomen, bloating, even fatty food intolerance do not prove that the gallbladder is at fault or needs to be extirpated. Many chapters in this book consider conditions that are mistaken for gallbladder trouble. The important ones to consider are ulcer disease (usually duodenal ulcer), antral gastritis (including the currently interesting condition of *Helicobacter pylori*), parasitic disease, and most commonly irritable bowel syndrome.

Postcholecystectomy Syndrome: What Is It?

When patients continue to complain of upper right quadrant pain after gallbladder surgery, they are often given a diagnostic label, *postcholecystectomy syndrome,* to account for the fact that they are still experiencing discomfort and the operation was unsuccessful. Some of these patients had little reason to have their gallbladder removed; they probably complained of discomfort that mimicked the typical colic attack, but clear evidence from tests was not forthcoming. Other diseases or disorders, the most frequent in my experience being irritable bowel syndrome, were probably to blame. Some, far fewer, have had a surgical mishap; stones left over in the common duct may remain silent for years at a time, only to kick up later. This problem can be determined and is a most satisfying diagnosis, since removal of the stones by a variety of techniques will solve the problem.

For some, the trouble is the fact that the surgeon left a portion of the cystic duct when removing the gallbladder in an effort to avoid ruining the common bile duct. A stone may have formed or be left over in this cystic duct stump (as it is called), and its removal should clear up the problem nicely.

Biliary Dyskinesia

When we have been unable to prove that your pain and discomfort in the upper right quadrant comes from disease of the gallbladder and have scraped the bottom of the diagnostic barrel (ruling out diseases like duodenal ulcer, pancreatitis, duodenitis, gastritis, and esophagitis), we at last consider the possibility that we are dealing with a "functional" disorder of the gallbladder and its ducts. Almost in despair of helping you, we raise the possibility that the trouble is the result of a discoordination or disruption in the flow of bile from the gallbladder, and the main bile ducts (*Figure 8*), caused perhaps by a spasm of the gatekeeper muscles at the end of the duct—the *sphincter of Oddi* (where the main pancreatic duct joins the main bile duct). To this still somewhat nebulous concept is given the name *biliary dyskinesia.*

Since functional disorders can and do occur throughout the entire gastrointestinal tract, from the esophagus on down to the rectum, there is no reason to believe that the biliary part of the GI tract *could not* also experience similar problems. The real test is *how* to prove it.

First, we must be sure that there is no mechanical reason or problem in the duct system, such as a leftover stone or a stricture or scar at the lower end of the duct. If this is a serious possibility, and blood studies at the time of pain do not give us evidence of obstruction, then it is now customary to examine the duct system by ERCP. This abbreviation stands for quite a mouthful: *endoscopic retrograde cholangiopancreatography* (see *Figure 6*)! The procedure involves the endoscope through which a rather thin tube is passed into the bile duct and dye injected. The risk here is that we may stir up the adjacent pancreatic duct and cause an attack of pancreatitis. By no means is this a trivial matter; it may occur in perhaps 2 to 3 percent of patients. So one thinks twice, or even thrice, before doing

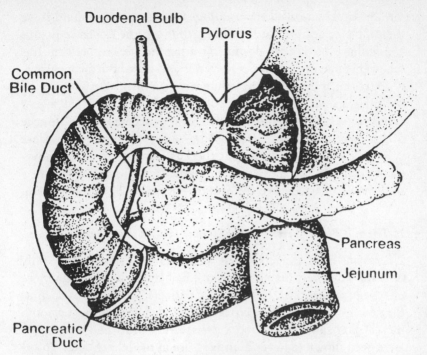

Duodenal Bulb

Pylorus

Common
Bile Duct

Pancreas

Jejunum

Pancreatic
Duct

FIGURE 8. Diagram of the relation of the duodenum and the pancreas.

or allowing the procedure to be done on one's patients. Yet most individuals tolerate ERCP well and do not have any serious side effects. When the ERCP has found no organic disease, then the possibility arises that we may be dealing with a functional condition in this region, where several fluids and two ducts make up an intricate plumbing system.

A lot of ingenious effort has been devoted to measuring the pressures in the duct and sphincter muscles. Biliary manometry can be done with appropriate devices, just as pressure measurements can be made in the sphincters of the esophagus and rectum. But biliary manometry is more difficult for the investigator, and for the patient. The hope with these studies is that we will find abnormal pressures and *then* confirm the possibility of dysfunction of the sphincters. If this train of thought is correct, then cutting the sphincter, an operation called *endoscopic sphincterotomy* should solve the problem; however, it is difficult to prove the existence of this condition. Most centers do not have the facilities to perform this type of manometry, and the reported results have been inconclusive. It does seem at times that the sphincter is cut in an effort to help the patient who has not responded to any other treatment. I would certainly be reluctant to recommend this procedure in the absence of any objective evidence. It is also possible by using a radionuclear scan—the HIDA—to show that there is some delay in the movement of bile through the bile duct into the duodenum. This may be a useful piece of evidence to confirm the suspicions of your physician.

Is There a Place for Drug Treatment with Biliary Dyskinesia?

It is reasonable to expect that, as we come to understand more fully how the sphincters function, we will be better able to design more effective medications to benefit our patients. Medications such as the newer calcium channel blockers, effective on spasms of smooth muscle that surrounds blood vessels of the heart and esophagus, have been shown to lower high pressure in the biliary duct. Unfortunately, this has not been studied systemically by researchers, but I have had some good luck with a few patients who have tried the calcium channel blockers; these individuals had found no relief with other medications and even sphincterotomy. But the whole area remains a no-man's land—or should I say, a no-woman's land, since women seem to have a greater tendency to fall into this diagnostic bin.

In addition to remembering that other disorders can produce discomfort and pain on the right side of your upper abdomen, we must avoid falling into the trap of blaming the gallbladder for belching, burping, and intolerance to fatty foods. These symptoms, long associated in the minds of both doctors and patients with gallbladder trouble, are not always, indeed not frequently, connected with that organ. Patients and doctors find, to their dismay, that removal of the gallbladder does not influence these specific symptoms. On the other hand, in this "stone age," perhaps we do not have the necessary techniques for studying functional aspects of the gallbladder in the absence of stones. There is the suggestion that patients who are receiving CDCA or UDCA to dissolve their stones have seen some improvement of their indigestion or dyspeptic symptoms, but not the bad pain from their colic. Perhaps the change in the chemical composition of their bile is having a good effect, but I do not advise the routine use of these bile acids for indigestion and fatty food intolerance on this slight evidence.

I have titled this chapter "The Gallbladder in the Stone Age" with more in mind than a pun. Our current thinking about the gallbladder and its problems is becoming more sophisticated and we are entering a modern epoch moving beyond a single simplistic mechanical approach to that organ.

At present, our only partially successful effort to prevent attacks of gallbladder colic, where stones have been demonstrated, is to reduce the fat intake in the diet of our patients. But it is clear from our preceding discussion that the problem starts with the liver making an abnormal bile. I see future efforts directed at correcting this defect before it leads to gallstones in the susceptible population. Genetic or biochemical tools I believe will make this goal science rather than science fiction.

9

When the Silent Pancreas
Speaks Up

The pancreas, a key digestive gland, sits unobtrusively in the upper back portion of the abdomen. It plays its part in digesting our food and preparing it for absorption so quietly and effectively that in health we never hear from it, let alone know it is there. When it is disturbed, it lets us know in no uncertain terms.

We can visualize the pancreas as a very active chemical factory, actually, two chemical factories housed in one building. The major portion of the pancreas is composed of glands that manufacture the digestive enzymes (*amylase* to digest starch, *lipase* to break down fats, and several other enzymes, *trypsinogen* and *chymotrypsinogen* among them, to digest the proteins). Synthesized for external export for use in the intestinal tube, these ferments move through the pancreatic ducts—the tubular pathways of the organ—and enter the upper intestine alongside the tube of the common bile duct, which comes down from the gallbladder and through which the gallbladder empties its bile. Remember, the bile is formed by the liver and is stored in the gallbladder between meals (see *Figure 8*).

In some individuals these two channels—the main pancreatic duct and the common bile duct—form one channel just as they exit into the duodenum. This is called the *common channel*. In most instances they flow alongside each other, in parallel fashion, emptying through a small mound called the *Papilla of Vater*.

Within the pancreas, scattered throughout the gland and especially numerous in its tail (the left side of the gland, which is furthest away from the duodenum), is another set of active chemical engines, the *Islet of Langerhans*. These specialized cells, clumped together in groups, form compounds that enter the blood for internal use elsewhere in the body; these are *internal secretions,* the hormones, the chemical messengers of the body. The most imortant of these is *insulin,* which regulates the blood sugar level and sugar metabolism; insulin deficiency causes diabetes. The islets are active protein factories that produce several other hormones as well: *glucagon,* which raises blood sugar; *somatostatin,* which turns off our intestinal juices; *vasoactive intestinal polypeptide* (VIP), which turns off the stomach juices, silences the gallbladder, and stimulates the intestine to secrete fluid.

From this brief overview of pancreatic function, you can appreciate that anything which inflames the pancreas, or destroys its cells—external and internal—or replaces them with new growths will disrupt this beautifully organized system.

The pancreas leads such a sheltered life in our abdomen that even aging, which reduces the efficacy of the stomach, has practically no effect on the working of the pancreas; however, this organ is very sensitive to the action of certain drugs, alcohol, caffeine, and trouble in the nearby gallbladder. Despite its importance in the normal processes of digestion and food absorption, the pancreas does not contribute all that much to ordinary forms of indigestion; yet it can cause trouble and show itself in two main ways, which depend upon the speed and intensity of the disturbance: in an acute explosive form, known as *acute pancreatitis,* and in a slower more insidious form, known as *chronic pancreatitis.*

The Not-So-Silent Pancreas

The most dramatic and rapid malfunction of this organ is known as *acute pancreatitis*. This is an acute inflammation of the pancreas. The usual scenario involves an otherwise healthy individual of any age and either sex who suddenly experiences upper abdominal pain, often starting in the middle, above the belly button, and spreading across to each side of the abdomen. Sometimes, there is pain in the middle of the back, since the pancreas sits across the upper back portion of the abdominal cavity. The pain can vary from mild to quite severe and can double the subject over, making him or her lean forward in an effort (usually futile) to get more comfortable. There may also be fever, chilly sensations, and sweating. At times, the inflammation may be minimal and cause only mild discomfort, which might be passed off as just another episode of indigestion.

But there are several other scenarios in which, at times, this frightening episode can occur. In women, a history of several pregnancies, a crash weight-reduction program, a family history of gallbladder disease or of gallstones especially in the mother or gallstones in the patient herself may set the stage. In this scenario, an hour after an indiscreet meal of fatty foods, which she ordinarily avoids, or after eating some delicacies at a party, the patient develops the kind of pain I have just described. In another typical episode, a man with an innocent past medical history decides to entertain some business associates at dinner in town, has a large meal along with a few cocktails, and precipitates a painful attack.

Harder to puzzle out is the subject who experiences acute pancreatitis and forgets to tell his physician about medication that he takes on an irregular basis. But this episode can also occur with medicines or drugs taken on a regular basis; the patient may simply forget to report them. Such an individual is often a woman who takes water pills, or diuretics as we physicians call them, from time to time because she retains fluid or wants to avoid the symptoms of premenstrual syndrome. Although taken only at specific times of her cycle, they have been known to cause acute pancreatitis.

In contrast to the almost volcanic eruption of acute pancreatitis is the effect of *chronic pancreatitis*. This term implies continuous low-grade persistent inflammation and scarring of the pancreas. This form may show itself in a number of different ways. *Pain* is the most common symptom, again in the same region of the abdomen as in the acute form, but usually not as explosive. This form is more persistent and insidious, and the patient often needs and receives increasing doses of narcotics for the pain, which may wake him from sleep in the middle of the night. In another, at times *painless* form, the symptoms reported by the suffering individual are quite different: appetite may be good, but weight loss occurs because the fats of the diet are not being properly digested and stored; calories are thus lost in the stools, sometimes but not necessarily with diarrhea. The undigested fats in the intestine, acted on by resident bacteria, may lead to some nausea, occasional foul belching, lots of gas, with passage of air through the rectum. Finally, if the islets have been involved in the inflammation, there will be trouble in handling sugars. Even the full picture of *diabetes* may develop, although there is no family history of the disease.

What Causes Pancreatitis?

There are many probable causes of pancreatitis, almost too many to be plausible. The problem is how to relate these causes to the resulting inflammation of the gland. But it is possible to visualize what is going on during an attack of pancreatitis. Imagine a number of triggering mechanisms set into action the digestive enzymes within the gland itself. They are stored in a kind of protective shell, or inactive form, and go into action where and when they are needed in the intestinal tract, where they begin digesting the food we eat. In *pancreatitis,* these digestive enzymes are suddenly activated and released within the pancreas itself and begin digesting the entire gland, so that the organ undergoes a volcanic eruption of sorts, scattering a host of toxic substances into the circulatory system, and thus throughout the body. It is these substances, often derived from proteins, that are responsible for the shock, a fall in blood pressure, fever, and the prostration that can accompany a severe attack. On the other hand, as I have indicated, many episodes are usually of lesser intensity and may be so mild that they are overlooked.

What Triggers the Autodigestion (Self-Digestion) of the Pancreas?

By far the two most common causes are (1) alcohol and (2) biliary tract disease. The first is more frequent in men and the second in women. These facts have been known for some time, although we are far from understanding precisely how each of these mechanisms damages the pancreas. We know, for example, that wood alcohol (methyl alcohol), if ingested by accident, causes a severe form of pancreatitis that results in hemorrhaging within the organ. I believe that alcohol acts as a direct poison on the gland.

A small group of patients with pancreatitis suffers from metabolic disorders, either *hyperparathyroidism* (overactivity of the parathyroid gland, which controls the level of calcium in the blood) or *hyperlipidemia* (an abnormal amount of lipids—that is, fat—in the blood). This group also includes patients suffering from the effects of diabetic coma. Occasionally, pregnancy or kidney transplantations may be complicated by acute pancreatitis. Also, *hypothermia*—that is, the accidental exposure to very low temperatures—especially among alcoholic and homeless people, has been known to bring on acute pancreatitis. Among the infectious causes of pancreatitis, several viruses have been implicated—mumps, the virus of infectious mononucleosis, and the Coxsackie-B infection.

Especially intriguing are the drugs that cause acute pancreatitis. They include such diuretics (water pills) as chlorthiazide (Diuril®), furosemide (Lasix®), and chlorthalidon; and antibiotics such as sulfonamides, salazopyrine (Azulfidine®), and tetracycline. High-dose estrogens have also been implicated, especially in women with hyperlipidemia. Other hormones that have been associated with pancreatitis include the adrenal steroids (cortisone and its derivatives), ACTH (the adrenocorticotropin of pituitary origin), and several immunosuppressive drugs, such as Azathioprine (Imuran®) and 6-Mercaptopurine (Purinethal®). With all of these drugs, the common assumption now accepted is that in some way or other these substances convert the inactive forms of the pancreatic enzymes into their active forms within the gland with prompt autodigestion of the organ taking place.

How Is the Attack of Acute Pancreatitis Diagnosed?

The most important thing that can lead your physician to recognize that your discomfort or severe pain is due to pancreatitis is to suspect it, to consider it as a possibility. Too often the milder forms of this disease are overlooked. The acute cases are usually more easily recognized. On physical examination, there is tenderness in the abdomen and occasionally the patient is jaundiced because bile flow from the liver or gallbladder is partially blocked by the swollen pancreas.

A simple test, and the most widely used, which will incriminate the pancreas measures the level of *amylase* in the blood. Ordinarily, the blood level of amylase has a well-defined limit of normality; therefore, each laboratory must determine the limits of its method for measuring it. Usually, in the normal individual, a mixture of amylase from various sources is secreted into the blood by the liver, the salivary glands, and the pancreas; the abnormal high level of amylase in acute pancreatitis, however, comes from the pancreas which spills its enzymes into the blood when the gland is inflamed.

The other pancreatic enzyme that can be measured in the blood is lipase, which you will recall splits fat. This too reaches high levels in the acute patient. The blood amylase and the blood lipase complement each other. Amylase usually appears earlier in the blood than lipase and may leave the bloodstream earlier. Lipase, however, remains detectable in the blood for a longer period. At times, your physician may in fact miss the peak measurements of both enzymes.

Nowadays imaging techniques reveal the state of the pancreas and adjacent organs, especially the gallbladder and liver, and are routinely used to document the diagnosis of acute pancreatitis, detect its complications, and shed light on its causes. The sonogram of the upper abdomen and the CAT scan can tell us if the gland is swollen and its surrounding areas inflamed. These methods can also find out whether there is trouble in the gallbladder because of gall-stones or obstruction to the flow of bile. A plain X-ray of the abdomen, without any contrast material such as barium, often reveals a paralyzed loop of the intestine adjacent to the inflamed pancreas called a *sentinel loop* and can show whether the pancreas has been the seat of trouble before. Calcification in the gland, in the form of stones in the pancreatic ducts (the tubes that carry the pancreatic juices to the intestine) or a "snowstorm" of calcium scattered throughout the substance of the gland, can indicate earlier attacks of inflammation that have gone undetected.

Treatment for Acute Pancreatitis

The *immediate* treatment for an acute attack of pancreatitis, which may require hospitalization in many instances, is outside the scope of this book, but it includes resting the pancreas by stopping all food by mouth, support of the circulation by adding intravenous fluids and blood components, drainage of the stomach and intestine through a tube inserted through the mouth or nose, antibiotics, and at times surgical intervention.

The *long-range* treatment following recovery from an acute attack requires long-range planning. We must search for causes and plan dietary reforms that will modify the patient's eating habits and perhaps even lifestyle.

The Search for the Causes of Pancreatitis and Prevention of Recurrence

Most important is the need to find a cause for a particular patient's acute episode of pancreatitis in order to prevent recurrence. The major cause in most male patients is alcohol and alcoholism. Recurrent attacks and chronic pancreatitis are thus prevented by avoiding alcohol. There is no alternative, unfortunately, and we all know how hard it is to treat alcoholics.

For the other major cause, gallbladder disease, the surgeon's removal of this organ may be rewarded by cure. I have already discussed the details of this procedure in Chapter 8. For the search to be thorough, your physician should order standard X-rays to detect the shadows of calcium-containing gallstones, as well as sonograms of the upper abdomen; CAT scans and MRI are less helpful. At times, the old-fashioned oral cholecystogram, a dye by mouth, and the intravenous cholangiogram may be useful in pinpointing the problem. These methods are described in the chapter on testing (Chapter 3). I have also discussed the use of duodenal drainage, to check for cholesterol crystals in the duodenal bile, in Chapter 8.

One must consider, too, the value and safety of the other available methods for visualizing the biliary tree, especially those used to detect the presence of stones in the common bile duct, including, of course, the ERCP (endoscopic retrograde cholangiopancreatography) discussed in Chapter 3 in the section "Liver and Pancreas." There is no question that ERCP is useful in that particular search, but one must bear in mind the significant risk of stirring up a recurrence of pancreatitis by employing this technique, especially in a subject who has recently had an acute episode. ERCP is also helpful when it is used to visualize the pancreatic ducts prior to considering a surgical attack on the chronically inflamed gland. It is most useful in planning any surgical correction of obstructed flow in the passageways of the pancreas and in assessing the amount of damage to the remaining portions of the pancreas. But here, too, ERCP runs the risk of inducing acute inflammation in the already chronically inflamed gland.

If the cause of the pancreatic attack has not been found through these standard methods, the search will require detailed detective work, including tracking down any medical information the patient may have forgotten to tell his or her physician or has concealed, as for example, alcohol dependence. A call to your pharmacist may help you collect the necessary information for your doctor. Obviously, any drugs that could have precipitated an attack are discontinued for good.

The metabolic diseases are usually easily detected by appropriate blood tests, but the presence of hyperlipidemia (increased fats in the blood) may be missed, particularly if you are examined at a time when you have not been eating or have been on a rigid low-fat diet. The metabolic causes can be corrected and, if successfully managed, no further recurrent attacks will occur.

Individuals with gallbladder disease can be treated by removal of the gallbladder, which will eliminate further pancreatic attacks. The variety of options available today are discussed at length in Chapter 8. The difficult problem of finding a cause, however, is very evident when you realize that probably 10 to 25 percent of patients do not fit into any clear diagnostic pigeonhole.

Treating the Impaired Pancreas

The pancreas has great recuperative powers that can restore it even after a severe attack. The individual who has recovered from pancreatitis need not suffer any chronic disturbance in digestion or metabolism, provided that no further damage is done to the gland again. If repeatedly insulted, however, by alcohol, undiagnosed gallbladder disease, toxic drugs, or uncorrected metabolic diseases, the pancreas will develop two serious difficulties.

1. The impaired secretion of insulin may lead to *diabetes* which will require the newer oral medicines for this disease or the use of insulin.
2. The impaired secretion of pancreatic juices and of its enzymes, needed to digest our diet, will lead to *weight loss*—in the presence of adequate intake of calories and in the event that your physician has placed you on a low-fat diet in order not to overtax the pancreas.

This latter difficulty can be corrected if the missing elements of the pancreatic juice are replaced by using any one of a number of available potent pancreatic enzyme preparations that contain the necessary enzymes, especially those for digesting fat. Usually in capsule form, these pancreatic replacements will need to be taken along with your meal—at the beginning, during, and at the end of the meal. Furthermore, the enzyme will have to be protected from being digested by the stomach's mixture of acid and pepsin by the use of histamine II blockers, which are described in Chapter 5. The use of pancreatic enzyme replacements can also control pancreatic pain by reducing the secretion of juices from the impaired gland.

Warning: A Too Easy Diagnosis of Pancreatitis

Acute, recurrent, or chronic pancreatitis is a serious condition, but it is too often invoked for anyone whose upper abdominal indigestion and discomfort do not easily fit into the common diagnostic categories. This is especially the case if a blood study reveals a modest rise in amylase. In my experience, a level slightly above a particular laboratory's normal is too often used to label the individual as having pancreatitis and further testing for other disorders is abandoned.

There are normal variations in the amylase levels in the blood that have no abnormal consequences. Furthermore, other organs—especially the salivary glands, liver, and fallopian tubes—can also contribute to the amylase levels (ordinarily little amylase is secreted from the normal pancreas into the blood). Before an individual is diagnosed as having pancreatitis, the amylase levels must be quite high (in the many hundreds or even thousands of units). Equally important, the diagnosis is strengthened if the lipase of the blood is elevated at the same time. Yet I have seen a number of individuals with both enzymes elevated who do not appear to be sick.

It is now possible to measure the different kinds of amylase in the blood by identifying what is called the *isoamylases*—that is, the circulating forms of amylase that resemble each other. In this way, abnormal amounts of pancreatic amylase can be distinguished from the amylase that originates from other organs, and the diagnosis of pancreatitis can be made with reasonable certainty.

It will help to put the information I have been detailing about pancreatitis in this chapter into the proper perspective if you will remember that most individuals who have an attack of acute pancreatitis usually do not go on to the chronic form. They recognize the wisdon of reforming their eating habits: reducing their intake of fat, especially animal fat (red meat, eggs, butter, and cream), and controlling their social drinking of alcohol. Eliminating any drug capable of triggering an attack and correcting any underlying gall-bladder disease will further ensure the complete healing of the inflamed pancreas.

10

Jaundice

Where Does the Yellow Come From, Where Does the Yellow Go?

This book is not a textbook of medicine and certainly not a textbook on liver disease, but the occurrence of jaundice is a dramatic event in any individual's life. It causes unusual symptoms and raises questions about the health of three large digestive glands associated with the upper gastrointestinal tract: the liver, the gallbladder, and the pancreas.

Simply, jaundice refers to the yellow color of the skin and the whites of the eye that results from the presence of the pigment bilirubin. This is the pigment that gives our bile its yellow-greenish color.

The yellowish tint of the eyes and skin may be very faint and difficult to detect because its intensity increases very slowly. In fact, those close to us, especially those who see us every day, may fail to notice this subtle transformation. However, someone seeing us after an absence may be struck by our complexion. It may be especially hard to recognize this pigment change under electric light, which is often rather yellow; reflective sunlight reveals the condition more easily.

Where Does the Yellow Come From and How Does It Get into the Skin and the Whites of Our Eyes?

Bilirubin is the end product of the breakdown of the pigment haem. This pigment is found mostly in the red cells of your body, but a little comes from muscles. Certain specialized cells scattered throughout the body chew up the haem, which results from the daily wear-and-tear on our red blood cells, and convert the haem to the yellow pigment bilirubin. For the body to get rid of this waste product, the albumin in our bloodstream carries the bilirubin to the liver, which transforms it so that the original pigment can become water soluble and be excreted from the body in the bile. You will recall that the bile is stored in the gallbladder. Bilirubin is finally dumped into the intestine through the bile ducts and then eventually out of the body in the stool. Some of the pigment worked over by the bacteria of the colon gets absorbed back into the blood and finds its way out of the body in our urine.

This process is going on all the time. There is always a small amount of bilirubin in our blood—less than .5 mg percent. But when larger amounts of bilirubin are formed or the machinery for getting bilirubin out of the body breaks down, the blood level rises and the pigment—bilirubin—gets deposited all over the body. It usually requires a rise of four or five times the baseline to be detected in the skin, the whites of the eyes, or the urine. The color of the skin and the whites of the eyes results from the yellow bile deposited in them.

How Is Jaundice Detected?

Recognition of jaundice depends simply on someone observing that an individual's skin and eyes are yellow. The person with the condition may not be aware of this. Often the earliest sign that someone is becoming jaundiced is observed in the darkening of the urine, which contains an increased amount of bile. Sometimes, the stools may appear lighter in color if the jaundice results from a process that blocks the movement of bile from the liver and gallbladder to the intestinal tract. Occasionally, if a blood sample is drawn because a person does not feel well, the increase in blood bilirubin may be found long before any skin changes are detected.

Why Is It Important to Verify the Diagnosis of Jaundice?

There are two main reasons. First, jaundice is striking evidence that something has gone wrong with a carefully programmed process that regulates the excretion of this waste product. Second, jaundice itself brings its own symptoms and discomforts. The most disturbing symptom, which can make an individual frantic at times, is intense itching of the skin. This discomfort can drive the sufferer to make deep, painful scratches in the skin. Often one's sense of taste is disturbed, and one's appetite—the desire to eat—falls off. Cigarette smokers lose their desire to smoke. But this loss of appetite for food and tobacco may result from the process responsible for the jaundice rather than the jaundice itself.

What Causes Jaundice?

It is obvious that any number of things can go wrong and result in jaundice, but they can be easily organized into three main groups of problems:

1. Increased load of bilirubin in the blood—a larger load than the liver can handle.
2. Disturbances in the liver itself that interfere with its work of getting the bilirubin into the bile.
3. Disruption or blockage of the path the bile must take from the liver or gallbladder to the intestine.

A hereditary defect in bilirubin metabolism or an increase in the rate of destruction of the red blood cells (due to immune mechanisms or a mismatched blood transfusion, for example) called *hemolysis* accounts for the first problem.

The second group, which must be carefully distinguished from the third, is due to disease of the liver itself: usually the result of viral infections, the effect of some drugs, and especially alcohol.

For the third mechanism, the common denominator is *mechanical blockage of the duct system of the liver and gallbladder,* which leads to obstruction by way of infection, inflammation, stones, tumors, or injuries to the duct (see *Figures 3, 7,* and *8*).

You can consider these three mechanisms as occurring (1) before bilirubin gets to the liver (pre-hepatic), (2) during the passage through the liver (hepatic), and (3) after passage through the liver (post-hepatic).

In Chapters 8 and 9, which discussed disorders of the gallbladder and pancreas, we saw how stones can cause infection and block the common bile duct. The inflammation of the pancreas, as well as tumors of this organ, can also obstruct the flow of bile.

A Common, Harmless, but Confusing Form of Jaundice: Gilbert's Syndrome

On occasion a perfectly healthy person with a perfectly normal liver, gallbladder, and pancreas may be found to have more than the normal amount of bilirubin in his or her blood when a sample is drawn for some entirely different purpose. From time to time the individual may even display a slight yellowing of the whites of the eye.

This condition is called *Gilbert's syndrome* after the French physician who first observed it. It occurs in about 2 to 5 percent of the population and results from a harmless inherited defect in the way the liver processes bilirubin. The important point is that it is not due to liver disease. Patients are often alarmed because they are suspected of having hepatitis. Occasionally, these individuals may have some discomfort after being exposed to other types of infection, and in the fasting state, they may experience some nausea or, at times, some discomfort over the liver area. But this does not represent liver disease. Those who have inherited this syndrome need to educate themselves about it and inform their physicians about it as well. They need to know that the jaundice may become more obvious after any current infection or if they fast or skip meals.

How Are the Different Kinds of Jaundice Sorted Out?

Jaundice due to excessive destruction of red blood cells is fairly easily recognized by standard blood studies.

The problem of separating those primarily due to the liver from those due to obstruction of the flow of bile into the intestine may be more difficult, since obstructive jaundice can lead to inflammation of the liver. This separation is of the utmost importance since relief of the obstruction will solve the problem of the jaundice and prevent liver damage.

Fortunately our current imaging techniques help immensely. Indeed, the first thing most physicians do after recognizing the presence of jaundice clinically or from blood tests is to order a sonogram of the upper abdomen (see Chapter 3). This will quickly reveal whether or not the tributaries of the bile ducts are blocked, and whether the pancreas is swollen. If need be, a CAT scan (Chapter 3) can resolve the problem further in pinpointing the site of obstruction to bile flow. On occasion one may have to follow this with an ERCP (see Chapter 3) which visualizes the bile and pancreatic ducts by injecting dyes into them which then can be recorded by X-rays.

Primary involvement of the liver as the cause of jaundice can be suspected from the initial blood studies of liver function, the history of medicines taken by the patient, and especially by blood studies of the variety of viruses that cause hepatitis: Hepatitis A, B, and now an easily available test of Hepatitis C, as well as a history of exposure to infected food, especially seafood, blood transfusions, or invasive surgery.

The important point is that jaundice due to obstruction requires prompt action: removing the obstruction, usually a gallstone, if at all possible, or bypassing the obstruction if the obstructing factor, a tumor or inflammation or scar, cannot be removed. (The surgical approach to gallstones is discussed in detail in Chapter 8.)

While these methods of deciding what the individual with jaundice is suffering from are being pursued, there are useful ways of relieving the sufferer's severe itching. Antihistamines (Benadryl® or Cholor-Trimeton®), some sedatives such as Atarax®, and the bile binder, cholestyramine (Questran®) are very helpful. Cholestyramine works by binding whatever bile may get into the intestine, and this in turn lowers the level of bile salts in the blood and tissues, which are the causes of the itching.

Fortunately jaundice is not frequently or usually associated with the majority of conditions that cause the dyspepsia or indigestion which this book describes, and our modern imaging techniques help make the diagnosis relatively simple.

11

Malabsorption and Maldigestion

Internal Starvation

To obtain the nutritional benefits of our diet, two complex processes must take place in an orderly fashion. First, the intestinal tract must *digest*—that is, break down—the complex foods we eat into the smallest part. Then the intestinal lining cells must *absorb* these parts across the intestinal wall so that the bloodstream can convey them to the tissues.

Before we turn to maldigestion and malabsorption, we must clear the air by eliminating and defining the question of *malnutrition*. Individuals may have many digestive symptoms, particularly loss of weight, as the result of under-nutrition—that is, simply not eating enough.

Depression, loss of appetite, loss of a sense of taste and smell, bad teeth, poor eating habits, poor food quality, and food fads can all lead to a reduction in food intake. This is *malnutrition*. We are not talking about this condition in this chapter. Individuals with maldigestion and malabsorption usually have good appetites. They lose weight because their bodies are starving in the presence of plenty, not because they are not eating enough.

How Do I Know If I Have Malabsorption?

When we suffer from such symptoms as bloating, belching, distention, and upper abdominal pain, we can easily understand that this discomfort stems from problems in digestion. But when is the question of malabsorption raised? The key symptoms of most malabsorptive problems are loss of weight (for adults) and failure to gain and grow (in children). You are eating the same daily diet that you have done for a long time, but now your scale shows that you are not only failing to stay in the same place, but have begun a slow, steady loss of weight. This is principally the result of a failure to absorb the calorie-containing fats which are lost in the stool. Sometimes people experience diarrhea, but not always. Indeed, the stool may contain lots of fat without being loose; often they are frothy, bubbly, with an oily sheen. We used to think that the stools in malabsorption float because of the fat content; but it is now known that they contain much gas and air.

The person suffering from malabsorption may also develop overall weakness because of anemia, which lowers the red blood-cell count (these cells contain oxygen-carrying hemoglobin). Anemia may result from a difficulty in absorbing iron in the duodenum, folic acid in the jejunum, or vitamin B12 in the ileum.

Malabsorption can also lead to mild spontaneous bleeding from the nose or rectum, and this bleeding often enters the tissues, giving the appearance of black and blue bruises without our having suffered any bruises or injuries. This occurs because the amount of prothrombin—a clotting factor manufactured in the liver from vitamin K—is lowered in the blood. It is the failure to absorb the fat-soluble vitamin K which is at the root of this problem. Occasionally, your fingers and toes may go into spasm—this is called *tetany*—because your blood contains low amounts of calcium, which in turn is based on your failure to absorb vitamin D (another fat-soluble vitamin). At times, you have pains in the bones of the spine or hips, or even a waddling gait, because your bones have become soft (a condition called *osteomalacia,* which differs from *osteoporosis,* a weakness of the calcium-containing salts of bone, seen most frequently in postmenopausal women and known to all of us through countless stories about it in newspapers and magazines). Finally, there may be swelling of the ankles, which has nothing to do with trouble in the heart. This swelling, called *edema,* is caused by a lowering of the albumin of our blood, either because we really are not absorbing our dietary protein well or we are leaking protein from abnormally leaky cells in the intestinal lining.

How Does My Physician Discover I Have Malabsorption?

First, your medical history is always the most important clue. Bring notes when you visit your physician, including your weight on specific dates, a history of intestinal operations that may have altered the normal traffic in the gastrointestinal tract, a family history of inflammatory bowel disease or celiac disease in childhood or family members, and perhaps a history of similar weight loss some time ago during your teenage years.

The doctor's examination may reveal some obvious physical signs: the pallor of your eyes or palms, evidence of easy bruising, possibly the swelling of your ankles, but often the physical examination does not add much information. Apparent skin disease—especially scleroderma with its thickening of the skin—is a very good clue that points to intestinal problems.

Will I Need Many Laboratory Tests?

Some simple blood studies will quickly point to malabsorption. They can measure the blood count to detect and analyze the anemia and the blood levels of albumin, calcium, and prothrombin. These tests will point your doctor in the direction of considering and pursuing malabsorption.

Once the question of malabsorption is clearly on the table, it must be settled if at all possible. A gastrointestinal series of X-rays of the entire gut (from mouth to the colon) will reveal if there are any gross disorders responsible for malabsorption. At the same time, specific blood and urine tests will help to pinpoint the defect in absorption. Blood level of carotene is a good general screening test for absorption, while the d-xylose test measures your ability to absorb sugars.

Examination of the stool for fat is the clincher for documenting caloric malabsorption, but the messiest test to carry out. There is no use measuring the 24-, 48-, or 72-hour output of fat in your stool unless you are taking a good amount of fat in your diet. It is a nuisance to collect all stools you pass through the agreed-upon period. For some physicians, examining the smear of a casual specimen of stool and staining it for fat under the microscope is a good simple shortcut.

For malabsorption resulting from a failure to handle milk and milk products, the current focus is on lactose (the sugar of milk). The lactose tolerance test—similar to the glucose tolerance test for diabetes—is very popular. In this test, the blood level of glucose is measured after you ingest 25 grams of lactose, thus providing evidence of whether you can digest lactose. I rely on the patient's history of milk intolerance for the most part. Moreover, as I have been emphasizing throughout this book, examination of the stool for blood and parasites is a standard procedure that should be part of all gastrointestinal investigations.

There is one more invasive test that may be needed to document adult celiac disease—also called *gluten enteropathy* or *sprue*—which accounts for adult malabsorption and an inability to digest the protein of wheat, rye, oats, and barley—that is, gliaden or gluten. For this procedure, a tiny piece of the lining of the upper small bowel is obtained through a biopsy instrument swallowed by the patient. If the subject is properly prepared with normal blood-clotting factors in place, the risk of this procedure performed as an outpatient is minimal and, in my opinion, one that a prudent person would take. I advise this test because if the specific finding of villous atrophy (that is, atrophy of the lining cells), the hallmark of sprue, is present, then you must remain on a gluten-free diet indefinitely (which probably means for life).

What Are the Common Causes of Malabsorption?

The basic defect that links together the various forms of malabsorption lies in the failure of the intestinal lining cell to function normally. The easiest case to understand is the individual who has had a large portion of the small intestine removed by an operation, no matter what led to the operation: inflammation of the wall as in Crohn's disease, or gangrene of the gut due to a blood clot, or just a simple twist due to an adhesion or band. This shortened or "short bowel" cannot be expected to absorb normally.

If the wall of the intestine is altered by disease, this, too, will necessarily interfere with the intestine's absorptive function and capabilities. These diseases include the inflammatory condition of Crohn's disease, tumors such as lymphomas or Hodgkin's disease, or damage caused by radiation.

In other instances the cause is in the biochemical apparatus of the intestinal lining cell. Some are hereditary—for example, the lack of an appropriate enzyme in the wall. In the case of lactose or milk intolerance, the enzyme is lactase. Some result from a defect in the lining cell that we don't fully understand, such as the inability of the body to handle a specific protein. In celiac disease, which can strike both infants and adults, the cell is unable to handle the protein gluten. But sometimes parasitic infestations can cause inflammation and lead to similar disruptions.

In short, just about anything—diseases, drugs, or radiation—that can interfere with the normal function of the intestinal lining cell can bring about malabsorption. The list does seem endless and calls for some extensive investigation and shrewd guesses by your physician to decide which trail to follow to reveal the particular malabsorptive syndrome you have.

But without calorie loss—that is, weight loss—you are not likely to have a true malabsorptive problem.

How Can the Usual Forms of Malabsorption Be Corrected?

Lactose intolerance can be handled by reducing the intake of dietary lactose. For children and some adults, the problem can be solved by adding lactase, Lactaid® now commercially available, to the dairy product. If you still are having trouble on a relatively low-lactose diet, you will have to be more vigorous in your search for food substances that contain small amounts of lactose, such as prepared foods (french-fried potatoes, pudding, pie fillings, dried foods, soups, instant potatoes) and drug tablets and capsules which contain lactose as fillers. If you have difficulties in handling sucrose, the sugar composed of glucose and fructose, this sugar will have to be eliminated from your diet.

From the point of view of calories, malabsorption of fat is much more important than malabsorption of sugar and proteins, so a shift in dietary intake in the direction of increasing carbohydrates and protein in the diet, with a simultaneous reduction in fat, may be temporarily helpful. But one needs to eat a lot more sugar and protein to make up for smaller amounts of fat. Medium-chain triglyceride (MCT), available as an oil (Portagen®), can help as well, since it is absorbed more easily than the long-chain fats in our normal diet, which include corn, olive, and palm oil.

Gluten enteropathy—or sprue—can be handled by simply eliminating gluten from the diet. For most sprue patients, eliminating wheat, rye, oats, and barley does the trick; all other foods may be eaten. The elimination of wheat is most difficult for patients, since bread, wheat cereals, pasta, and so many other foods must be avoided; however, the rewards are gratifying. Occasionally, a sprue patient may need to eliminate lactose as well as chicken and eggs, and, very rarely, a patient displays, inadequate pancreatic secretion and requires pancreatic enzyme replacement. Also on rare occasions, an individual may require steroid therapy with its attendant risks, but the soon to be introduced, rapidly eliminated steroid could be substituted for prednisone.

The serious inflammatory condition of the small intestine known as Crohn's disease can be treated today with a variety of medications and, if the problem is localized, by surgical resection of the diseased area.

If bacterial overgrowth is present because of unabsorbed sugar, starch, or fat, and this plays a part in the patient's discomfort, an antibiotic directed against the intestinal invaders is often helpful in eliminating gas, which can be foul at times, along with abdominal distention, bloating, and cramps.

Maldigestion or Malabsorption?

Distressing intestinal symptoms can plague us when we fail to digest our food properly (*maldigestion*) or when properly digested food fails to be absorbed into our bodies (*malabsorption*). Bloating, belching, gas, diarrhea with cramps, all these may develop, often creeping up insidiously. Symptoms may even go beyond the digestive tract. A person may experience weakness, bruise easily and without apparent cause, and bleed from the mouth or gums.

Maldigestion

I began this chapter by distinguishing *malabsorption* (failure to absorb our diet) from *maldigestion* (failure of the gastrointestinal tract to break down the diet into its constituent parts).

If you recall Chapter 1, which discussed the intricate functioning of the digestive tract, you can easily appreciate how things can go wrong if the digestive glands in the wall of the intestine, or the pancreas, or the liver fail to split our diets down to the small pieces which can be absorbed. We may eat a good, wholesome, and well-balanced diet with plenty of protein, carbohydrates, and fats, but, if they are not broken down as they should be, we will simply lose their nutritive value as they exit from the gut and never get deposited in our tissues. It's as if we make a deposit in our bank, but our bank statement never records it.

Carbohydrate and Starch Maldigestion

The long-chain sugars that make up the carbohydrates and starches of our diet require the enzyme amylase for digestion, but can be broken down even without the salivary gland's contribution of amylase. Things will go wrong, however, if the pancreas, at a later stage of digestion, does not pour forth the required amount of its *amylase* into the intestine. *Pancreatitis,* the inflammation of the gland (either acute or chronic), or *tumors* (growths in the gland), which either block the exit passages of the pancreas to the intestine or replace the normal glandular tissue, can prevent starches from being broken down or digested (in our strict use of the word). The disease *cystic fibrosis,* if present in the pancreas, can cause carbohydrate maldigestion in children because the pancreas does not secrete the appropriate amount of amylase. Even if the pancreas can make enough starch-splitting enzymes, its task may be overwhelmed if the stomach empties its load of carbohydrate too quickly into the upper intestine; thus stomach operations for ulcer disease or bypass operations for obstruction can lead to carbohydrate malabsorption.

Aside from amylase, lactase and sucrase are two additional enzymes needed to break down sugars. Lactose, the sugar present in milk and other dairy products, requires the enzyme *lactase*. This enzyme functions in the wall of the intestine and breaks lactose into glucose and galactose. Sucrose is present in cane sugar and the fruits of our diet, and requires the enzyme *sucrase* to break it into glucose and fructose. If deficiencies in these enzymes are present at birth, they are likely hereditary. If, however, enzyme deficiencies become evident in adult life, they probably result from disease of the small intestine, which may partially or completely destroy the enzyme-producing cells. Acute inflammations and viruses, bacteria or parasites, nutritional disorders such as sprue, inflammatory conditions such as Crohn's disease, or injuries resulting from drugs or X-rays can contribute to enzyme deficiencies. So you can see that it is difficult at times to distinguish maldigestion from malabsorption because they are closely linked in sequence.

A very rare difficulty is the patient who cannot handle mushrooms because of a deficiency in the enzyme *trehalase* that digests *trehalose*, a carbohydrate of that food. This deficiency is also hereditary.

Fat Maldigestion

I pointed out earlier that the fats in our diet (the triglycerides) are broken down into their constituent fatty acids by the fat-splitting enzyme *lipase* secreted by the pancreas with the aid of bile salts secreted by the liver. The fatty acids are then rearranged into micelles (small droplets coated with materials which make them soluble), which can cross the intestinal wall into the body.

Obiously, diseases of the pancreas (inflammation, tumors, congenital malformations) disturb this orderly process. In addition, micelles may have trouble forming if there is a problem in getting the proper amounts of bile into the intestine, which would result from obstruction to bile flow due to stones, scars, surgery, or tumors. If the body does not recycle the bile because of disease or malfunction in the ileum, then it may lack the necessary amount of bile salts needed. Finally, the bile salts may not function properly because their composition is disturbed by the presence of colonic bacteria which invade the upper small intestine.

Protein Maldigestion

There is a large, built-in safety factor in protein digestion that makes protein maldigestion rather rare. Even in the total absence of the *pepsins* in the stomach, protein digestion proceeds normally unless a very large portion of the pancreatic protein-splitting enzymes are absent. This requires extensive inflammation (pancreatitis) which usually results from excessive alcohol, blockage of the ducts due to stones, or tumorous growths.

Treatment of Maldigestion

I have just catalogued a variety of disorders that contribute to maldigestion. Here I want to call your attention to several ways of coping with the problems of maldigestion.

For example, we can replace the gastric pepsins, pancreatic lipase, and the pancreatic protein-splitting enzymes, especially trypsin, with potent forms of these substances that have been extracted from animals and are now commercially available in varying and competing forms.

Bacterial overgrowth can be reduced and controlled by judicious use of antibiotics directed toward the common inhabitants of the lower gastrointestinal tract. Bile salts can be given by mouth in several tolerated forms.

Dietary management may also be very helpful in the instances of maldigestion. Since fat maldigestion causes the most loss of calories and thus of weight, the diet can be shifted to one higher in carbohydrates and proteins, thereby reducing the fat content. Finally, the medium-chain triglycerides—usually referred to as MCTs—unlike the long-chain triglycerides of our normal diet, need not be converted into the micellar form to be absorbed. Thus MCTs can be given in place of the usual fats in the diet as a nutritional supplement.

12

Food Intolerance and Food Allergies

"Was It Something I Ate?"

Those who have read my previous book, *Your Gut Feelings,* may recall that I titled the chapter on this subject "Food Allergies: Fact or Fancy?" Since then, more has become fact and less fancy, but a great deal remains to be discovered about this common and puzzling problem.

Indeed, it is difficult to know exactly how many individuals suffer from food allergies. The estimates range all over the lot. *USA Today* recently stated that 60 percent of the population has a food allergy. The Asthma and Allergy Foundation states that about 1 percent of the entire American populace is allergic to food; while the U.S. Department of Agriculture guesses that the number is between 10 and 15 percent.

All too often we use the word *allergy* loosely. After a meal that has made us uncomfortable, we take for granted that some food "doesn't agree with me." When we experience nausea, belching, burping, indigestion, dyspepsia, or heartburn, in the upper abdomen or lower chest, followed by diarrhea and cramps in the lower abdomen, we declare, "I must be allergic to something I ate."

At times, we explain our gastrointestinal distress by claiming that we cannot tolerate this or that drink or food, and yet at other times we can eat and drink the same foodstuff without suffering any unpleasant reactions. We know that hay fever sufferers do not always sneeze when pollens are floating around because their threshold varies from time to time with the height of the pollen counts.

Can we sort out these differences? In all this loose talk and thinking can we find some definite facts?

No one doubts that food allergies exist, but because controversy and possible quackery surround the whole subject, doctors approach it with great caution. The major problem is that it is difficult to prove that the symptoms blamed on food allergies are really caused by foods. Common symptoms include (1) gastrointestinal ones (nausea, vomiting, abdominal cramps, diarrhea); (2) distant symptoms (hives, swelling of the lips and throat, known as *angioneurotic edema,* and eczema); (3) asthma and swelling of the nasal passages; and (4) migraine. With such a diverse list you can see why your doctor might feel defeated even before beginning an investigation of possible causes.

Another reason why food allergies are difficult to identify is that the diagnostic tests are hard to interpret and unreliable. For example, *skin tests* in which extracts of the suspected foodstuffs are either pricked or scratched into the skin are widely used and equally widely suspected because they are unreliable. Recently, a great deal of energy and money has been spent on detailed chemical analyses of hair and fingernails in an effort to relate these findings to presumed nutritive deficiencies arising from disturbed diets. Although some understanding of the body's nutritional status, especially protein balance, can be gained from hair analysis, most of these expensive tests shed no real light on the nutritional causes being studied. Another group of tests, including radioallergosorbent tests (RASTs) and the measurement of immunoglobulins of the blood, especially immunoglobulin E (IgE), have a better scientific foundation but are expensive and often inconclusive. As a result, patients, physicians, and nutritionists resort to *elimination diets*. Either specific foods (e.g., milk) or classes of food (e.g., wheat or dairy products) are forbidden or a few simple foods allowed and new foodstuffs gradually added. The elimination diet approach is widely used but difficult to follow given the daily demands placed on the actively employed individual.

Finally, food allergies are tricky to diagnose because the different kinds of reactions to food need to be separated and better defined. Recently, clinical researchers have made a start in this direction in an attempt to upgrade the scientific bases of the classification of these reactions.

So it is not surprising that the general public and those who suspect that they have food intolerances or allergies feel frustrated. Jane E. Brody, the noted and respected personal health columnist and science writer for the *New York Times,* in its magazine section of April 29, 1990, speaking for the public and for herself, raised the important question about the growing controversies in this field, asking if doctors are paying enough attention to the problem.

Terms: Getting the Categories Straight

Food intolerance, the most widely used term, covers the whole gamut of adverse reactions to foods and includes the two main groups: *food idiosyncrasy* and *food allergy.*

Food idiosyncrasy refers to a specific reaction to a specific food substance, perhaps based on a specific defect in the body's enzyme system. *Phenylketonuria,* a disease in which the newborn infant cannot handle a specific amino acid and which is tested for routinely at birth, is such an example.

Food allergy refers to an adverse reaction to food that satisfies two criteria: (1) the participation of a component of the immune system (often quite difficult to prove), and (2) the recurrence of symptoms on two or more occasions when the suspected food is retested.

However, it is often very difficult to decide whether an allergic factor is present even if you react badly every time you eat a specific substance. This gray area can include drugs as well as food. Aspirin sensitivity is a good example. The fact that some individuals react to aspirin with asthma or eczema suggests that an allergy is present, yet the mechanics that cause the reaction have not been shown to be immunological.

Food intolerances that occur every time an individual eats or drinks a specific substance may be due to a direct chemical toxic effect. Rapid heartbeat after consuming tea, coffee, chocolate, or cocoa may result directly from the caffeine, theobromine, and methylxanthine in these substances.

With lactose intolerance, for example, individuals experience bloating, "gas," abdominal cramps, and even diarrhea after drinking milk or eating dairy products (e.g., cheese, ice cream, butter). Still other individuals, as they grow older, may develop these reactions to milk, although they did not experience them earlier in life. A considerable part of this intolerance to milk is due to the presence in milk of the sugar lactose (composed of one molecule of glucose and one molecule of galactose), which is split and digested by the enzyme lactase, present in the cells lining the intestinal tract. The lack or reduction in the amount of lactase leads to some of the unsplit lactose reaching the colon, where the intestinal bacteria feed on it and produce gases and irritating acids. Lactose intolerance is now widely known by the general public. Those who need to drink milk can partially correct the lactase deficiency by adding a special enzyme preparation to the milk. Lactaid® is one such available remedy. The difficulties some people have with milk may also be related to other substances it contains, especially proteins. Milk contains at least 20 proteins and these can cause true allergic reactions.

Other substances such as wine may induce reactions, because toxic materials are released when they are left to stand around after being opened. Foods that contain histamine, such as fermented cheeses and sausages, or that contain histamine-releasing tyramine, such as chocolate, cheeses, and canned fish, can also produced reactions that mimic allergic reactions.

Another food intolerance most people have heard of is the Chinese restaurant syndrome. Characterized by gastric distress, warmth, flushing, headaches, and dizziness, this reaction is presumed to result from monosodium glutamate (MSG) contained in

Chinese dishes. Symptoms often appear within 30 minutes after eating.

The additive and preservative sulfites can cause reactions that have led to wines and other products being labeled as containing them.

As you can imagine, the list of foods suspected of causing allergic symptoms is long. In one study of 100 patients, the following foods were tested for sensitivity; the number of individuals claiming sensitivity to the food is given in parentheses: milk (46), eggs (40), nuts/peanuts (22), fish/shellfish (22), wheat-flour (9), tea and coffee (8), chocolate (8), artificial colors (7), pork/bacon (7), and chicken, tomatoes, soft fruit, and cheese (6 each).

In a more recent report, another group of about 200 individuals who could identify a specific food intolerance were tested; the following percentage of individuals complained of these foodstuffs: cheese, 35 percent; onions, 35; milk, 34; wheat, 30; chocolate, 30; butter, 25; yogurt, 25; coffee, 24; eggs, 23; nuts, 17; citrus fruits, 18; tea, 18; rye, 18; potatoes, 15; barley, 13; oats, 12; corn, 11; alcohol, 7; fruit, 8; yeast, 6; vegetables, 6; red meat, 4; salads, 2; spicy foods, 2; additives and saccharin, 2; bran, 1; and fat, 1.

Products that contain mold spores may also be a problem, and these would include highly aged cheese, wine, yogurt, and yeast.

True Food Allergies

Experiencing symptoms such as swelling of the lips or tongue, a runny nose, hives, asthma, or eczema, within minutes of eating a certain food, is clear evidence of an allergic reaction.

If your symptoms begin more than an hour after eating the suspected food, it is more difficult to prove that they are caused by an allergy. The first thing to do is to be certain that these symptoms recur every time you eat the suspected substance. In addition to the symptoms mentioned above, those that may appear more than an hour after a particular food is consumed include such gastrointestinal effects as vomiting, diarrhea, abdominal pain, bloating, and constipation. In rare cases, intestinal bleeding may be caused by an allergic mechanism. To rule out an intestinal disorder that can cause the same symptoms, your doctor should first take a careful history, give you a complete physical examination, and request all the appropriate laboratory tests.

Wheat Intolerance

Wheat or substances that contain the wheat protein called gluten, such as wheat-containing flour, bread, cakes, stuffings, pasta, and so on, appear frequently on the list of substances people cannot tolerate. Gluten is present also in rye, oats, and barley.

One disease, *sprue,* or *gluten enteropathy,* as it is technically labeled, is a form of intestinal malabsorption that is clearly due to the inability of the individual's intestinal lining cells to handle gluten. This leads to malabsorption, weight loss, loss of fat in the stools, and often diarrhea and bloating. A chronic skin condition, *dermatitis herpetiformis,* also known as *Duhring's disease,* may also be associated with sprue or spruelike changes in the small intestine. The striking point here is that removal of gluten from the diet leads to prompt restoration of health and disappearance of symptoms. The diagnosis rests not only on the good effect of withdrawing gluten from the diet, but on the fact that biopsies of the small intestinal lining reveal marked abnormalities that return to normal as the individual's health improves. In a few cases, people with sprue need to remove lactose from their diets as well. Very rarely, even removal of these two major offenders is not enough, and other substances such as chicken and eggs must be eliminated from the diet.

We still don't know whether the sensitivity to gluten in sprue is purely an allergic (immunologically mediated) reaction or is also in part a toxic reaction. Before the discovery in the 1960s of wheat's role in sprue, this disorder was treated with cortisone to suppress a presumed immunological inflammation in the intestinal wall.

MILD WHEAT INTOLERANCE

Unlike sprue, mild wheat intolerance does not inflame the cell lining of the intestine, but it does cause intestinal symptoms such as bloating, gas, distention, and even diarrhea. There is no laboratory test to prove this condition, only the reactions of the individual to repeated attempts to eat wheat or wheat-containing foodstuffs.

Although almost everything we eat that is digested by the intestinal secretions is completely absorbed by the body, some starch is not broken down by the appropriate enzymes, escapes absorption in the small bowel, and reaches the colon. The amount varies from individual to individual and depends on the kind of starch. For example, the carbohydrate of rice flour is absorbed completely, whereas some of the carbohydrate of all-purpose white wheat flour is not. This malabsorption in some individuals can be corrected by withdrawing gluten from the diet.

This curious phenomenon is thought to be caused by an interaction between starch and wheat protein, which interferes with the former's complete absorption and thus produces unpleasant gut sensations. Until we understand this problem better, however, it is important not to fall victim to the many untested remedies that have been proposed, such as eating certain substances with only certain other substances; you risk developing a lopsided diet.

How Do We Diagnose Food Allergies and Intolerances?

The first step in deciding whether your intestinal symptoms are due to an intestinal disorder or a food intolerance is for your doctor to eliminate those intestinal disorders and diseases that can cause identical symptoms. If this has been done, and you or your family have a history of allergies (such as eczema, hives, allergic asthma, or runny noses), it's more likely that your intestinal symptom is caused by a food allergy.

As noted at the beginning of this chapter, it is difficult to make a clear-cut diagnosis of food allergy; skin tests, for example, are unreliable. Your medical history is, of course, terribly important, especially if you can recollect the specific circumstances of an "allergic" episode. For example, a dramatic intestinal explosion following your consumption of strawberries or shellfish will never be forgotten! Memory is not always reliable, however, so we have come to rely on the old standby—*elimination diets.* Tedious, boring, and difficult as they are to carry out, especially by busy people on the move, elimination diets offer the best way to diagnose a food allergy. If you undertake such a trial by diet, you will need to follow it religiously, keep detailed notes, and not give up after a few days. I believe any elimination diet must be followed conscientiously for at least two weeks.

Although your doctor may have his or her own recommendations, I suggest eliminating one and only one of the most common offenders at a given time: milk, wheat, egg, spices, perhaps nuts, especially peanuts. For milk, it is not enough to switch to skim milk. You must eliminate all milk and milk-containing products, such as cheese, ice cream, yogurt, and butter. For cheese, there is no substitute, although recently an ice cream substitute containing tofu has become available. Nondairy creamers can be substituted for some of milk's uses. Margarine is a good substitute for butter, but you will need to look at the label closely to see that the product you select does not contain any milk solids (in the United States, Fleischmann's margarine is one such product).

If the elimination of one of these common offenders does do the trick, your future course is clear: you must eliminate that entire class of food from your diet. Because some reactions depend on the dose of the offending food, you might be able to tolerate a small amount. You will have to determine this yourself by careful testing.

What if these simple elimination diets do not help? If a few conscientiously followed trials do not work, you must consider the possibility that you do not have a dietary problem, especially if a full diet doesn't make you feel any worse. If you and your doctor are convinced that food plays a part in your distress, however, there are a few more tedious trials and trails that you may want to follow.

One option is to go on an *elemental diet,* the kind of diet the astronauts have tried. These are expensive, not very palatable, prepared diets that are chemically pure. Vivonex® is one such commercially available elemental diet, Flexical® another. Because they are quite unpalatable, most people are unwilling to stick to them, but they are worth considering.

A more acceptable, although still difficult, approach is the *core diet*. For about 20 years I have recommended this very restricted, though simple, diet to those concerned that their troubles are dietary. Only four substances are allowed in as many meals as you wish, and it's a good idea to stock up enough of each to last for two weeks:

1. *Bottled mineral water*.
2. *One starch* (either rice or potato but not both). (Instant rice or raw rice [white or brown] can be cooked with the mineral water.)
3. *One meat* (either boiled, broiled, or roast chicken without the skin, or broiled lamb chops, but not both).
4. *One canned fruit* (I suggest Bartlett pears).

It is extremely rare for anyone to be sensitive to these few substances. This diet should be followed for at least two or preferably for four weeks until your intestinal turmoil subsides; only then can one new food be added every other day, with egg, wheat, and milk as the last to be added. If a new addition produces a reaction, you "back up" to the previously tolerated level and start in again after a week of stabilization.

You can see how this can be tedious and rather cumbersome to carry out, but some well-motivated individuals have been able to pinpoint the offending food or foods with this approach. I should warn you, however, that allergies of this type are not common.

British investigators have suggested we try a slightly less rigorous starting or core diet, especially in patients with an irritable gastrointestinal tract. In one study, their recommended tests lasted three weeks, with strict attention to the diet. They had their patients exclude dairy products, cereals, citrus fruits, potatoes, tea, coffee, alcohol, as well as foods containing additives (difficult sometimes to know with so many prepared foods) and preservatives. Moreover, these researchers also excluded any food the patient had already identified as causing symptoms. They allowed fresh meat, fish, vegetables, rice, and products derived from goat's or soy milk. In addition to a strict faithful follow-up on the diet for three weeks, all medicines the patient was taking—unless life depended on them—were stopped.

If the subjects had no improvement, they were told firmly that food and drugs were not causing their problems. One-half of the patients who carried out the program felt better. In the second stage of the study, participants added new foods only every two days before going on to another. If the symptoms returned, the offending food was avoided. The period of reintroducing the new dietary items was a slow process that lasted up to two to three months. About three-quarters of the patients were able to pick out one or more offending food substances. Most did well if they remained on the diet. Interestingly, about 50 percent identified two to five foods as upsetting them. These patients were mainly sensitive to dairy products and grains.

A point to remember is that one may suffer an adverse reaction to food after a viral or bacterial intestinal infection. Milk, eggs, and wheat may cause difficulties, but these problems are usually short-lived. The intestinal tract recovers and loses its sensitivity to these foods.

Can Medication Help?

The real cure for food allergies or food intolerances is the elimination of the offending substance. Lactase in the form of Lactaid® can help in lactose intolerance, but, in general, drugs are not helpful except to provide some symptomatic relief. Antihistamines of the two general types (benadryl and cimetidine) have not worked in my patients, and one would certainly not use any more powerful anti-inflammatory drugs. One drug that has been in vogue for immunologically mediated food allergy (IgE) is sodium cromoglycate (Cromolyn®), which is marketed abroad as the drug Nalcrom®, but my patients and I have been disappointed in its use. Although for a while the Letters to the Editor section of several good medical journals contained anecdotes of the effectiveness of this substance, submitted by doctors who were treating themselves, I would not send you abroad to get this drug. In the United States, it is available in capsule form as an inhalant for children with asthma, but the dose is far too small to be worth trying as a remedy to treat food allergies. The patient might need to take five capsules four times daily. This capsule also contains lactose, a substance the individual may be trying to avoid.

Let me conclude by saying that physicians are paying more attention to their patients' complaints of this kind. More good research on adverse reactions to food is being done. One does not need any clairvoyance to predict that the near future will lead to more facts and less fancy.

13

The Passage of Time

The Aging Upper Digestive Tract

In the United States, the fastest growing sector of the population is the 65-and-over age group, currently numbering about 28 million. Students of demographics project that by the year 2050 one out of every eight of us will be 75 years and older. We all experience the effects of age on our bodies, and can see its visible mark, but what does time do to the gut? I have discussed its effects on the lower intestinal tract in *Your Gut Feelings*. Here I discuss the upper gastrointestinal tract.

While age does make a difference, on the whole the structure and workings of the organs of the digestive system are relatively spared many dramatic effects of time, unlike the central nervous system and the cardiovascular organs.

The Mouth

The taste of our food and drink is perceived by the *taste buds* on the small protrusions of our tongue, called the *papillae*. As we age, the number of buds and papillae tend to decline, as well as the acuity of the taste buds. (The sense of smell is said to be the first sensory system to decline with age.) The salivary glands may also atrophy a bit with age and in later years may sometimes be unable to moisten the mouth. Because of these physical changes, some older individuals may lose interest in food and enjoy their diet less.

Swallowing and the Esophagus

Difficulty in swallowing, caused by problems in the upper throat, does increase with age and may result in malnutrition. At times, food and fluid may spill into the windpipe (the trachea) and lungs. This condition stems mainly from neurological and muscular disorders rather than the effect of time on the swallowing machinery. Strokes, diabetes, and Parkinson's disease are the chief culprits.

For a time, some difficulties in swallowing were ascribed to aging alone, and the term *presbyesophagus* was invented to describe the complaints. More recent studies, however, have revealed only minor effects of aging on the physiological movements of the esophageal muscles.

The Stomach and Duodenum

As we get older, our stomach makes less acid when empty and when stimulated. And while these findings are consistent with the changes that take place in the lining of the stomach, mainly thinning and atrophy, I doubt this change in the digestive process contributes much to the indigestion of the elderly.

When we turn to the question of age and the most common disorder of the upper gut, peptic ulcer, some puzzling facts emerge. First, while during the last two decades peptic ulcers and their complications seemed to be on the decrease, this did not hold true for the elderly. Particularly disturbing is the fact that there is an increasing number of gastric ulcers reported in women over 65 years of age and in men over 85. Yet duodenal ulcer does not seem to follow this pattern. Bloody, tarry stools (discussed in Chapter 5 on peptic ulcer) are the most often reported symptom of peptic ulcer in this age group. But many do not even have a warning period of pain. This is especially worrisome, since these individuals may have a bleed or have a perforation with serious outcome.

A second point is probably the most important thing we have learned in the last few years. It may be that the increased incidence of peptic ulcer is to be related to an increased use of nonsteroidal anti-inflammatory drugs (or NSAIDs, discussed in Chapter 5) in the older population as a remedy for arthritic pain. Of those taking these drugs, almost one-half are over 60 years of age, and about a quarter of their bleeds are associated with these drugs.

Earlier in Chapter 5 I discussed the possible use of the prostaglandin analogue Misoprostol and the efforts to prevent or minimize complications related to NSAIDs. Also discussed earlier is the emerging role of the bacterium *H. pylori,* which is among the most interesting current findings in ulcer disease, though the case has not been proven beyond a reasonable doubt. The presence of this "bug" in the human stomach increases with age, and it may be that the decrease of acidity with age or a damaged lining allows the organism to spread and thrive.

I should also call your attention to the side effects of our anti-ulcer drugs. In the older population, cimetidine can contribute to mental confusion. Constipation, so prevalent in the elderly, can be aggravated or caused by the aluminum-containing antacids as well. Diarrhea may result from the magnesium-containing antacids and from the prostaglandin-like drugs. These are points frequently overlooked since elderly patients take a great many pills and medications.

One last point deserves mention in our discussion of peptic ulcer therapy and the elderly. While we are now doing less surgery for ulcers, those who have had a part of their stomach removed for ulcer several decades ago can run into trouble with the passage of time. Those individuals who have been followed for more than 20 years following the operation have a greater risk of developing a tumor, even cancer, in the remaining portion of the stomach. If you are in this group, you need to be followed closely with our modern imaging techniques, which I have presented in Chapter 3.

The Pancreas

The pancreas has great reserves. Although the gland may show some increase in scar tissue or fat with age, it does not lose its digestive capacity with time. Perhaps its sheltered position gives it some protection.

The Gallbladder

Although more women than men have cholesterol gallstones, with age they increase in both sexes equally. The same holds true for pigment stones; men in earlier years experience more of these stones than women, but with age the incidence evens out between the sexes. Although the risks of an operation to remove stones from the gallbladder or ducts are greater in the elderly, it is here that some of the alternative techniques for managing gallstones (discussed in Chapter 8) will undoubtedly play an important part. A prediction of future trends in disease management is always risky, yet I believe that laparoscopic cholecystectomy (discussed in Chapter 8) will prove a very useful addition to our current methods of removing gallstones in the elderly.

General Nutrition

Loss of teeth, diminution in the senses of smell and taste (so important in the enjoyment of food), sedentary habits, even the boredom of eating alone after the loss of a spouse often conspire to induce poor appetite and therefore poor nutrition in the aging population. As a result, the consequent loss of weight often leads to the unsuccessful, medically fruitless search for serious underlying disease. It does not seem possible that individuals could develop scurvy in the twentieth century because of an inadequate intake of vitamin C in the form of fresh fruit, vegetables, and citrus juices, yet it does occur from time to time in the elderly. Certainly lack of adequate calcium intake contributes to the osteoporosis and weakness of aging bones.

With age, there can also occur the overgrowth of the small intestine with bacteria which ordinarily live in the colon. This in turn leads to digestive symptoms, interference with normal fat digestion, and even failure to absorb vitamin B12 adequately. Hydrogen breath tests with an oral dose of lactose are a simple way to detect this overgrowth, and the therapeutic response to intestinal antibiotics such as tetracycline is most gratifying.

14

The Brain–Gut Connection

Almost all patients, many stomach doctors, and everybody's grand-mother "know" that nerves can upset our gastrointestinal tract, making us feel sick and perhaps even contributing to serious dis-ease. We talk about the person who has no ulcer but who "gives" others stomach ulcers.

If philosophy, as someone once said, is finding better reasons for what we believe on instinct, then psychosomatic medicine may be considered the attempt to prove by scientific methods what we feel about the stomach on instinct. The belief that discomforts and dis-turbances of the gut arise from disturbances in our feelings and emotions has a long history. We know that fear can make a heart beat faster, dilate our pupils, dry our mouths, and loosen our bowels. This was known long before the term *psychosomatic* was coined.

What do we really know about this most important issue? Not very much, really. But our failure to prove the connection between our brain and gut does not prove the idea false. For example, we suspected for a long time that antacids healed duodenal ulcer, as well as relieved pain, but we had not proved it until recently. So we must avoid closing our minds and, above all, we must avoid being dogmatic.

Certainly, the machinery for getting messages from the brain to the upper gastrointestinal tract exists. There is the *rapid* transmitting apparatus of the central nervous system and its connections to the stomach, esophagus, and small bowel. There is also the *slower* apparatus of the hormones (chemical messengers) which allows information to be exchanged between brain and gut via the bloodstream. And there is new information that both of these systems can be influenced in turn by our immunological system.

As for the rapid apparatus, the nervous system of the intestinal tract—often called the *enteric nervous system* (ENS)—clearly is connected to the brain by the vagus nerve and by the sympathetic set of nerve fibers that emanate from the spinal cord. Some have seen this enteric nervous system as the "little brain" of the gut. Clearly, it is influenced by the real or "big" brain, but is not a real brain in itself since it probably does not store information, have a memory bank, or learn from experience. The ENS is more like a spinal cord in the wall of the esophagus, stomach, and upper abdomen that can send its messages back to the brain mostly through the vagus nerve, which carries the feelings of nausea and distention. Sensations of pain are carried through fibers that accompany the sympathetic nerves.

Until fairly recently, the connection between the emotional centers of the brain and the intestinal tract was believed to be solely by way of the connecting nerve pathways. Some recent discoveries about the chemistry of the brain, however, have caused a revolution in our thinking about how the brain communicates with the gut. It has been long known that the intestine communicates with different parts of itself or its attendant glands (liver, pancreas, gallbladder) by chemical messengers called *hormones.* These hormones are long chains of amino acids (the building blocks of proteins) known as *peptides,* which are assembled in specialized cells of the intestine (especially in the stomach and small bowel). The hormones released into the bloodstream signal intestinal muscles to contract, valves to open, glands to secrete water, acid, or bicarbonate, specialized cells to pour forth digestive enzymes, and the whole intestine to behave in a smooth, harmonious fashion.

Now, with the revolution in neuroscience, we have learned that these chains of amino acids, the *peptides,* are present in the brain and its far-flung nerves. These chemical messengers are not merely stored in the parts of the nervous system but are actually manufactured there. As a result, the nervous system not only transfers information within itself, but can also signal other parts of the body directly. Interestingly, each gland in the body usually manufactures its own special hormones. Only the thyroid makes thyroxine, for example, while the ovary makes its own distinct sex hormones. The brain and the gut, on the other hand, can and do make identical substances, and can thus "talk" directly to each other. The answers are far from complete, but it is becoming clearer how emotional disturbances, which lead to changes in the chemical activity of the brain, can in turn send disturbing messages to the gastrointestinal tract, and how the intestine in turn can "talk back" to the brain. We are beginning to understand how "brain feelings" can express themselves as "gut feelings."

An interesting example of a brain peptide that can affect the stomach—at least in animal models—is the brain-formed thyrotropin-releasing hormone (TRH). This chemical messenger from the brain increases acid and pepsin secretion in the stomach, increases blood flow to its lining, increases the muscular contraction of the antral portion of the stomach, hastens the gastric emptying of its contents, and facilitates experimental ulcerations in that organ. On the other hand, other chemical messengers from the brain—such as beta endorphin—produce the opposite effect. This polypeptide reduces acid secretion and gastric emptying contractions and prevents experimental ulcers. So one can imagine how ulcers might be driven by the balance and opposition of several chemical processes. The application of this kind of study to humans undoubtedly will follow as soon as our technology for measuring these minute substances improves.

The clearest example of a brain–gut connection is seen in the activation of the upper gastrointestinal tract at the start of a meal. The thought, the smell, the taste, the chewing and swallowing of food set off the appetite juices of the stomach even before the food reaches that organ. This occurs strictly by way of the vagus nerve. Since the nerves of the stomach contain not only fibers that relay sensation and can start acid and pepsin secretion, but also fibers that are the "start" and "stop" signals for the muscles of the walls of the stomach, it is easy to appreciate that the brain can lead to both inharmonious as well as smoothly synchronized contractions. Here is the anatomical and physiological basis for dysfunction of the stomach, and even the esophagus, which may originate in our thoughts and feelings.

The Role of Stress in Functional Indigestion

Before we consider the possibility that diseases may be caused by emotional upsets, what about the purely functional indigestion and non-ulcer dyspepsia for which all current researchers have failed to detect an organic cause? Many individuals' non-ulcer indigestion is part and parcel of irritable bowel syndrome (IBS), a condition in which the entire gastrointestinal tract is irritable, including the esophagus.

Victims of IBS are divided into two main groups. One group, usually selected and investigated, is made up of those who seek care and attention in hospital clinics and doctors' offices. A second, a vast group with similar symptoms, never attends clinics or seeks care for their symptoms. Those who seek medical care experience a great deal of uncomfortable anxiety, more than the control community population. The second group has no more psychological complaints than other members of the community. It does seem, on the basis of other studies as well, that those with IBS and dyspepsia who visit gastroenterologists experience more psychological distress than colleagues in their community. But there is an interesting difference between those with IBS and those with dyspepsia. Individuals with IBS suffer more from depression and mood swings, while individuals with dyspepsia experience generalized anxiety.

What seems to be emerging from this kind of investigation is that the psychological disposition or attitude of people sets a threshold for tolerating a wide variety of functional complaints. For reasons no one knows, certain individuals have a very low tolerance for functional changes in the GI tract from one end (the esophagus) to the other (the colon). This seems to hold for a wide variety of triggers—artificially induced stress under laboratory conditions, the natural stress of everyday life, reactions to food, and of course traumatic, catastrophic events in the personal life of an individual. Obviously, any method or technique that would enable us to handle stress better would certainly be of value in helping us to live more comfortably with these functional symptoms.

What Is the Role of Stress in Diseases of the Upper Gastrointestinal Tract?

One might imagine that the easiest stress-related disorders to investigate would be those in which stomach acid digests adjacent tissue—like the esophagus, duodenum, or the stomach itself. But these disorders are difficult to study. The very act of having a patient swallow a tube to collect and measure stomach acidity influences the level of acid. The most surprising finding of a great many studies is that strong emotions occurring spontaneously with painful stimuli or stressful encounters, or induced by them, usually suppress or inhibit acid secretion rather than increase it.

Perhaps we should be looking at the protective mechanisms in the lining of the upper gastrointestinal tract—meaning the whole list of agents which defend the lining from being attacked by acid, such as the secretion of bicarbonate, prostaglandins, mucus, and so on. At present, however, we have no evidence in this important area.

Earlier, in Chapter 5 on ulcers, I mentioned that, while all ulcer patients have some acid in the stomach, one-half of ulcer patients secrete normal amounts of acid. Thus it is hard to fit this evidence, too, with the idea that nervous tension leads directly to increased acid secretion and this, in turn, to ulceration.

Yet one cannot escape the many personal accounts in which ulcers, dormant for many years, suddenly flared up, bled, or even perforated under the stress of sudden tragic news. Or under other circumstances, some long continued irritating pressures finally "eat away" at our insides, as our friends or family have complained to us. So I, for one, believe that for some of us stress can aggravate ulcers through perhaps indirect pathways and chemical disturbances we do not yet understand.

On the surface, *gallstones* and *gallbladder colic* seem to present a different scenario. The formation of stones, secondary to the biochemical effects in the liver, appears so very remote from emotional origins and independent from our feelings and moods that it is difficult to connect their presence or occurrence with stress. Yet stones which the individual has known are there in the gallbladder for years will suddenly erupt and attempt to move out of the organ, not merely after a fatty meal or any obvious dietary provocation. One might speculate that the motor function of the gallbladder—its contractibility—can be influenced by nervous or hormonal triggers set off by stress; but this is still highly speculative. In Balzac's novels at least, characters can appear jaundiced after a severe emotional upset.

Pancreatitis, both acute and chronic, seems so closely tied to gallbladder stones in women, alcohol in men, and medications in both, along with disorders of calcium and fat metabolism that the idea of its relation to emotions or stress seems removed indeed. *Malabsorption,* especially the carefully studied gluten enteropathy (the sprue or celiac disease of adults and children), also seems so clearly biochemical or immunologically dependent that stress is not often invoked to explain the disease's ups and downs. Yet careful observers during the first half of this century were impressed by the link between celiac disease in adults and continued emotional turmoil. So perhaps it would be wise not to dismiss these older observations so cavalierly at present.

So Where Does This All Lead Us?

I cannot help feeling that when we use expressions such as "I cannot swallow what is going on in the office," or "So-and-so's behavior nauseates me," or "I cannot stomach X's carrying on," or "His feelings are eating away at his stomach" we are doing more than just using figures of speech. We are emphasizing the role of our feelings in altering our gastrointestinal tract and its behavior. We need no scientist to tell us that when we are depressed we lose our appetite and that when our children throw a temper tantrum they may vomit as a result.

The question of whether repeated disturbances in function due to a person's emotional state can lead to actual diseases of the gut has been a much harder one to answer. At present, there is no firm consensus among researchers. For much of this century a group of diseases was considered purely *psychological* in origin. These "classic seven" included peptic ulcer, high blood pressure, bronchial asthma, neurodermatitis, overactive thyroid disease (hyperthyroidism), ulcerative colitis, and rheumatoid arthritis, and each was supposed to go with a specific personality type. These "psychosomatic" diseases were believed to bridge the gap between functional disturbances and organic structural disease.

However, increasing experience and study have blurred this simple picture. The idea of specific personality types prone to develop a given disease did not stand up. The link between the psychological functions in an individual's life and the change in their tissues has not been demonstrated. Now emphasis has shifted from the emotional unconscious to the stress of everyday life. Scales have been devised to rate the degree of stress that major life events can induce, and investigators then try to correlate an individual's degree of stress with the severity of the disease.

Thus investigators in this field are not looking at stress for *the* cause of a disease whose origin is unknown, but rather trying to find out how stress influences the course of an illness, and to what degree. They are especially interested in how stress affects the medical or surgical program of treatment the person is following. In part, this shift in emphasis to stress and psychological aspects of illness reflects the widespread feeling that medicine has become too impersonal, too determined by high technology. We want our physicians to consider us as a whole person rather than as a collection of organs. This trend partly reflects the growing conviction that the investigative techniques of the neurosciences will help researchers make progress in putting the mind and the body together. As a result, the role of stress is no longer looked at only in those illnesses whose cause we don't know, but in all chronic illnesses.

In conclusion, there clearly is a brain–gut connection. Under normal conditions, this is a harmonious interaction which coordinates a complex and, as yet, poorly understood relationship. It is not difficult, therefore, to grasp that there may also arise at times, for a variety of reasons, a discoordination between brain and gut.

For the time being, then, I believe we can conclude that emotional turmoil and daily stress do play a part, along with our customary eating habits, the use of alcohol, caffeine, and tobacco, and our general lifestyle, including the amount of exercise we obtain, in how our entire gastrointestinal tract "feels" and its physical condition. The fraction each of these factors plays must be thoughtfully reviewed by both patient and physician. In such a careful analysis it may become apparent that for some individuals a consultation with a psychiatrist, psychologist, or psychotherapist is as much in order as the consultations with the gastroenterologist or the radiologist. Although I have not found formal psychoanalysis helpful for my patients, counseling that attempts to identify the real stresses of daily life and suggests ways of handling them has been of considerable use to them.

Many forms of relaxation techniques are now available, including taped instructions and formulated texts. Physicians now prescribe these in treating high blood pressure, sometimes before and along with dietary and drug treatments. There is a place for this approach in helping yourself to pinpoint stressors in your daily routine to try to get them under control.

Although I cannot entirely agree with the late Norman Cousins, who in his *Anatomy of an Illness* felt that his own serious immunological illness was cured by laughter and good humor, I certainly can agree that an optimistic disposition, a cheerful personality, and the cultivation of fun have tided many patients over the difficult course of their gastrointestinal illnesses.

The term *behavior modification* covers a whole host of psychological interventions used in counseling, suggestion, and self-hypnosis, which help individuals to alter and abandon their self-destructive habits and routines that dictate behavior, eating, and dependence on drugs, alcohol, tobacco, and especially painkillers. This approach, which focuses on altering present behavior rather than on understanding the past, can be very useful as well.

III

APPENDIX

In this Appendix, I want to discuss some mundane disturbances which are often upsetting to the individual and which at times are associated with the major conditions discussed in the preceding chapters, but not necessarily so.

Belching

We all know what a belch is: the sudden abrupt escape of gas into the mouth and throat, usually in a noisy fashion. A hiccup is quite different; it involves the spasmodic contraction of the diaphragm which forces gas out of the stomach and into the esophagus. A belch is the escape of gas from the stomach to the esophagus, and from there to the throat. I look at "burps" as just a series of little belches.

Mothers know that babies are often uncomfortable after being fed, especially if the baby has been swallowing a great deal of air during feeding. The infant is held straight up and patted gently on the back to make it easier for gas to escape from the stomach. Babies apparently need to be burped, but usually adults do not.

Much research has been applied to studying what happens during the reflux of acid from the stomach into the esophagus in an effort to understand heartburn. On the other hand, relatively little effort has been devoted to belching, but a few modern studies have begun to shed some light on this trivial, but often embarrassing, phenomenon. Key studies have shown that gas reflux—that is, reflux of gas from the stomach to the esophagus—is triggered by the distention of the stomach by gas or air. The gas exits the stomach when the lower muscular gatekeepers—the esophageal sphincters—relax; it is somewhat similar to what occurs when acid reflux takes place, in this case, in the lower sphincter, but not really dependent on impairment of the lower sphincter muscles' strength.

The last step in belching occurs when the upper esophageal sphincter relaxes in turn and allows the air in the esophagus to escape into the throat and mouth. Both these areas of relaxation are under the control of the vagus nerve. Relaxation and gas reflux occur more frequently when we are standing upright than when we are lying down.

Ordinarily, there is always some air in the stomach under normal conditions. When a plain X-ray of the abdomen is taken, the stomach bubble—the gas pocket in the upper half of the stomach—is easily noticed and invariably seen. Only those individuals with *achalasia* of the esophagus—also called *cardiospasm* (having nothing to do with the heart)—have no air bubble. Under normal circumstances, the gas bubble consists of (1) the air we have swallowed while drinking beverages and eating our food, especially if we talk while eating, (2) some of the gas contained in the carbonated soft drinks we Americans have such a passion for, and (3) the carbon dioxide which is released from the pancreatic juice that interacts with the hydrochloric acid of the stomach, a mixture made in the stomach and duodenum.

Most of us normally burp up some gas from our stomach and pay no attention to it. But when this occurs more frequently, we become annoyed. If the belch brings with it the gastric juices of the stomach, it may become painful and be associated with heartburn.

What Is the Significance of Belching?

Most of the time when we belch or burp, it has no serious significance. We are simply decompressing or lowering the pressure of the gas in the stomach. When the burp is associated with some pain behind the breastbone (heartburn), then it is part of a more complex reflux action that eases the pressure. Rarely, there may be some reason why the stomach fails to move its air and fluid contents on into the small intestine instead of back into the esophagus. Belching may thus be a clue to delayed gastric emptying, which we have dubbed *gastroparesis*.

Probably the most common form of belching occurs in the nervous individual who is talking and swallowing lots of air. For others, swallowing air while drinking hurriedly is more frequent; a cocktail party where one drinks and talks animatedly is an ideal situation in which to increase the chances of burping and belching. Smoking cigarettes or sucking on a pipe continuously also helps to increase belching.

Very frequently, burping is blamed on the gallbladder, which has in fact very little to do with the process. More often, because fatty foods seem to stir up belching, the gallbladder is wrongly blamed. It may be that fatty foods which relax the lower esophageal sphincter favor gas reflux.

Sometimes, when the lower intestine is filled with fluid and stool, pressure on the stomach makes us feel as if our stomach too is filled with gas. In these cases, we think we would feel much better if only we could burp up some air or have "a good hearty belch." At times, taking a small amount of carbonated water may help, but usually this simply perpetuates the sensation.

What Can You Do About Belching?

Belching is not usually a symptom of any serious disease, but it does indicate some things about your habits. Do you burp after every meal? Perhaps this is an indication that you are eating too hurriedly or talking while eating and swallowing air. Perhaps you are a smoker and suck on a pipe or a cigar throughout the day without giving it a thought. Then there are the many carbonated beverages we all consume that can overdistend the stomach. Minor burps and belches, however, should not send you to the medicine cabinet.

Nausea and Vomiting of Unknown Cause

There are countless and diverse reasons for our episodes of nausea, many of which do not concern us in this book. But it is a puzzling symptom which presents problems in treatment. There are individuals who have episodes of nausea that may at times lead to vomiting but in whom no general systemic disease exists; these are patients whose X-rays and endoscopic examination reveal no structural reason for their symptoms. As our methods become more sophisticated and specific hypotheses are tested and eliminated, we often have to admit we don't have the answers. Unfortunately, there is a growing group of patients, who also seem to complain of vomiting, along with their nausea. No small number of these sufferers wander from clinic to clinic, and from doctor to doctor, seeking some relief.

The idea is now emerging that these persons are suffering from a disturbance in motility—in the movement of the stomach and duodenal musculature. Equally important is the notion that this disturbance in motility—or *dysmotility,* as it is sometimes called—arises from disturbances in the electrical rhythms of the stomach muscles. These are dysrhythmias much like those we observe in the heart. We can measure the electrical rhythms of the heart on an electrocardiogram and detect minute disturbances of heart function through this device. Similarly, researchers are now pursuing methods of measuring the electrical activity of the stomach so that disturbances and abnormalities can be studied; unfortunately, none are yet routinely available for clinical application to patients. We now know, for example, that just as in the heart there is a normal pacemaker that times and initiates the electrical and muscular contractions of the stomach. This timekeeper exists in the body of the stomach, high up, near the fundus.

Disturbances in the rhythm of the stomach's electrical activity are of three types: (1) faster than normal, which is called *tachygastria;* (2) slower than normal, called *bradygastria;* and (3) a highly irregular activity, simply referred to as an *arrhythmia.* Tachygastria usually results from an ectopic (out of place) pacemaker abnormally situated at the edge of the stomach (the antrum). Bradygastria appears to arise from an abnormality in the normal pacemaker, which is found in the body of the stomach. The place of origin of the irregular arrhythmias is unknown. These dysrhythmias can be entirely innocent and cause no symptoms in some individuals. In others, they cause the unexplained nausea and vomiting we are discussing, as well as delayed gastric emptying and even abdominal pain. Drugs and circulating hormones can also induce these abnormal rhythms. Some experiments have shown that the substance prostaglandin E2, for example, can start an abnormal gastric rhythm; thus some individuals have been treated with medications that inhibit the formation of prostaglandins.

The whole area of dysmotility due to dysrhythmia is a most interesting and promising one; yet much at present remains mere speculation. We can surely expect progress as simpler methods of measuring the electrical activity of the human stomach are found and drugs developed to control the abnormal rhythm. Dilantin®, which dulls the electrical activity of the brain, has been used in an attempt to influence this type of arrhythmia, especially tachygastria, but there is very little in the way of convincing reports of its effectiveness. Inhibitors of prostaglandin formation such as indomethacin have been tried, but these substances can also inflame the stomach lining, and thus I would be reluctant to use them.

Dry Mouth and Bitter Taste

There are two complaints which many individuals suffer that are annoying to them and frustrating to their doctors. One of them is dry mouth, officially labeled *xerostomia;* the other is a bitter taste.

Dry mouth is a common enough complaint that one assumes results from failure of the salivary glands of the mouth to produce enough saliva. But this is not the case in most individuals and difficult to prove in others. Some medications can cause this condition: antidepressants are among the drugs which suppress saliva. The older anticholinergic drugs used in ulcer treatment, such as belladonna, atropine, or Pro-Banthine®, produce dry mouth along with other unwanted side effects. Less common causes are dehydration, previous X-ray treatment to the salivary glands, and the curious tissue-connective disease called *Sjögren's syndrome.* The sufferers of this disorder also have difficulty making enough tears and complain of dry eyes as well. They may require artificial teardrops as well as the artificial salivas I will discuss in a moment.

Dry mouth is very unpleasant and may be particularly disturbing at night if the individual is a mouth-breather. Many of these sufferers have trouble swallowing any dry foods and need to constantly swallow water during their meals. Other than helping with swallowing and digestion, saliva has several other useful functions. Mechanically, it helps clean the mouth by removing food particles and bacteria. It also plays a role in limiting dental caries. Dry mouth is said to predispose sufferers not only to dental decay but to fungal infections, especially thrush, which is linked to *Candida albicans.*

While such medications as pilocarpine can stimulate the flow of salivary juices, they are rarely effective in the day-to-day life of patients. If the problem is really vexatious, we must turn to artificial salivas. Most of those commercially available contain carboxymethyl cellulose or mucus as a lubricant, a sugar with low caloric content, such as sorbitol for flavoring, and water and salts to mimic real spit. The mucus-containing ones appear to be more effective than those containing carboxymethyl cellulose, but these artificial salivas are not terribly helpful. Unfortunately, their relief lasts for not more than an hour or two. Some people feel that sips of water do just as much for them, leaving patients unhappy and their doctors frustrated.

Bitter taste, or what is often described as a *bad taste in the mouth,* is a very common complaint plaguing a good many persons. The tongue looks quite normal when examined. The papillae—the tongue's little ridges—seem quite okay. Even when they are thinned out or atrophied, many individuals have no complaints. And, in fact, most patients with a bad or bitter taste in the mouth have no trouble tasting ordinary flavors. They recognize sweet, sour, salty, and bitter easily enough, but they identify "a bad," often difficult to describe, taste in the mouth all the time.

By the time they come to see a gastroenterologist, these individuals have had their teeth and mouth hygiene checked thoroughly by their dentist; they have no carious teeth, infected gums, or chronic tonsillitis, and no evidence that their sinuses are draining material into their mouths. Studies of the upper and, indeed, lower intestinal tract reveal no organic disorders. They have no food remaining in their stomachs to give rise to foul odors from bacterial activity. So why are they uncomfortable? Unfortunately, we have little to offer them. A few medicines, such as metronidazole, can give rise to a metallic taste, as if copper coins were placed in the mouth, but this taste is quite different from that experienced by these individuals. I am no psychiatrist or psychotherapist, but in most instances I have found this complaint to go along with others that suggest these individuals are depressed. Their lives, as well as their food, taste bad to them and help must be sought along psychological lines, which may include antidepressant medication.

Difficulty in Tasting

It is hard to separate the complaint of a "bad taste" in the mouth from a small and more specific group of patients who have *difficulty tasting foods and flavors.* The actual sensations created by food and drink seem to be missing in these individuals. I have seen this especially with a few older patients and thought I could detect atrophy of the taste elements of the tongue, although I have not done any scientific testing. Of those with this complaint, the largest group are individuals who have been treated with extensive courses of antibiotics and developed not a white-coated tongue, but a brown or even black tongue. This side effect will clear slowly with time and usually with full restoration of the whole range of taste sensations, once the tongue's coating is finally shed.

Much of what we consider the taste of food depends on our sense of smell. Nasal infections and chronic sinusitis can interfere with our ability to perceive odors and thus interfere with our sense of taste. Aside from this small minority, I have found little to explain the complaint except to pass it off as a symptom of "aging."

Some current research is being directed to improving patients' loss of taste sensitivity. A number of pharmacological agents can enhance taste perception (methyl xanthines found in coffee, tea, and chocolate, chemicals such as adenosine and inosine, and a cardiac drug, bretylium tosylate) but have little clinical application since they must be applied to the tongue for at least four minutes and have central nervous system and other systemic effects. Sometimes in despair I have advised a tablet of zinc (in the form of zinc sulfate, at 225 mg/day), which occasionally has a dramatic effect, but which may be purely a placebo reaction. Nonetheless, we can be grateful for some comfort, even though we may not always understand its mechanics.

A Lump in the Throat

Occasionally, during the course of a meal, or after it, or at times when we are not even swallowing, we experience a sensation we identify as "a lump in the throat." It is hard to explain what we mean to a doctor, but the sensation is clear and uncomfortable. We do not feel that food is lodged in our throat. We do not mean pain in the chest behind the breastbone, or heartburn, the burning sensation we all recognize. We simply have the sensation that there is a lump in our throat, and that is what we point to when explaining the complaint to our doctor.

Since X-rays of the esophagus or a look down the gullet with the esophagoscope usually reveals no mechanical blockage, this functional condition (which is *not* organic) was considered, at least when I was a medical student, as a nervous and neurotic trait. Indeed, the term *globus hystericus* was applied to the condition.

At present, we think differently about this condition. If you recall from Chapter 1 that the upper level of the esophagus is guarded by a gatekeeper muscle—the upper esophageal sphincter—you will remember this muscle may not act properly and fail to relax, or may at times contract forcefully with an increase in pressure. Sometimes barium X-rays that capture the act of swallowing will reveal the trouble. We can also measure the pressure across the sphincter and demonstrate the presence of spasms or increases in pressure. At times, however, these sophisticated techniques, including motion picture films of swallowing (cinéradiography) do not reveal any abnormality.

The important point here is that your doctor makes certain that no growth or mechanical obstruction is causing the sensation. In rare cases, a diverticulum, or outpouching, above the sphincter may be present. More frequently, spasm accounts for this sensation. In any case, we should avoid muscle-cutting operations in these areas. Sometimes simple antispasmodics or muscle relaxants help. Occasionally, the use of such medications as the calcium channel blockers, which relax the smooth muscle around blood vessels (particularly of the heart), can give relief.

Again, the important course of action is to be sure no organic disease is present and that no blockage exists. Once this has been established, doctor and patient can be reassured that nothing more need be done.

Butterflies

What about "butterflies in the stomach"? A common enough complaint we have all experienced before giving a talk, performing in front of an audience, or taking an examination is an uncomfortable fluttering that seems located in the stomach. For some individuals, it is a throbbing sensation felt in the upper abdomen. I have always interpreted this sensation as one coming from anxiety and probably related to rapid beating of the abdominal aorta, probably due to a surge of adrenalin into the system, akin to the tremor of the hands that some violinists suffer from before a concert. Drugs such as beta-blockers (Inderal®) have been reputed to help these performers, but I don't recommend them for "butterflies."

Difficulties in Swallowing

I want to discuss in this part of the Appendix several more serious complaints that individuals have that are related more directly to the problem of indigestion that we have been considering throughout this book. They include trouble in swallowing and delay in emptying the stomach.

Occasionally, we feel that our food is sticking in our gullet and point to a spot on our breastbone. It was only a momentary feeling and seemed to be related to the spongy consistency of the food we were eating, perhaps bread, or more often meat, but it did not cause us much discomfort. Sometimes a glass of water washed it down, so we paid it little attention.

But if this experience recurs and keeps on recurring, then it does become worrisome and we seek medical attention.

What Happens During Swallowing?

To understand what can go wrong in swallowing and cause us difficulties, we need to recall briefly what we covered in Chapter 1 on the workings of the upper gastrointestinal tract.

Swallowing is a complex, coordinated, and programmed act that requires the transfer of material from the mouth to the throat and involves the relaxation of the upper gastrointestinal (esophageal) sphincters. This swallowed material is moved along by the muscular contractions (peristalsis) of the esophageal muscles, which carry it finally to the stomach, once the lower esophageal sphincter is relaxed. Obviously esophageal swallowing can malfunction because of a *mechanical blockage* or because of a *functional disorder* of the muscular apparatus.

What Is Usually the Cause of a Malfunction in Swallowing?

Persistent difficulties in swallowing in the majority of individuals result from a structural problem in the esophagus: a mechanical blockage. Scars and growths are what we commonly suspect.

The scars or strictures are the result of inflammation, usually because of esophagitis, which is associated with the reflux of acid material from the stomach back into the esophagus (discussed at length in Chapter 4). In the young patient and one with a history of reflux and heartburn over the years, this kind of nonmalignant obstruction is most likely. If the individual is older, with no history of heartburn in the past and with very little discomfort, then we must pursue the problem promptly, which means X-rays and endoscopy, to be sure that no abnormalities exist, especially a growth.

What About Other Kinds of Difficulties in Swallowing?

I want to devote most of our attention here to those kinds of *dysphagia* (trouble in swallowing) which are not clearly related to a mechanical barrier—the kinds that are associated with indigestion, the kinds that are not revealed through endoscopy and in which X-rays may help very little. We are talking about the functional disturbances in the muscular action of the esophagus that cause discomfort and food to get stuck.

How Do These Muscular Disturbances Show Themselves?

I have already indicated that benign thick scars can be present in the younger person; this is also true for the muscular disorders of the esophagus. The symptoms come on slowly, rarely reveal a complete blockage when first reported. The discomfort in swallowing involves liquids as well as solids. But the esophagus can be cleared by taking liquids and with repeated acts of swallowing.

Sometimes the nature of the food that gets stuck and its temperature can shed some light. Meat and bread are frequent offenders because of their spongy consistency. Liquids, too, can cause trouble in this group. Cold drinks, for example, may aggravate the trouble by inducing spasm of the muscles, but hot drinks may relieve the condition somewhat, if only temporarily, by relaxing the esophagus. Sometimes individuals with muscular troubles in swallowing also have a history of heartburn as well as spasm. The area of the chest that the person points to, to indicate where the food is sticking, may not represent the actual place where food is being lodged, because it is not the *obstruction per se* that causes the pain, but the *stretching or distention of the esophageal tube* filled with material which causes the discomfort. Stretching, distention, and contraction of muscle are the most important causes of gut pain.

How Do We Know that Dysphagia Is Due to a Muscular Problem and Not a Structural One?

We do not begin to think about a muscular problem until the X-ray of the esophagus with barium and the endoscopic examination have reassured us completely that this organ is free of mechanical roadblocks. *I cannot overemphasize this point.* Obviously, we need to know that the sufferer does not have Parkinson's disease or has had a stroke, since a central nervous system disorder interferes with swallowing. Sometimes during the X-ray examination, the patient may be given some bread, a marshmallow, perhaps a bagel to swallow, and this may trigger and reproduce symptoms the patient is reporting.

What Is the Diagnostic Clincher?

At present, the most reliable method for identifying this group of muscular disorders is esophageal manometry. This procedure measures the pressure waves in the esophagus and the contraction and relaxation of the lower esophageal sphincters and guardian muscles—the gatekeeper muscles. This technique is described in detail in Chapter 3. Actually, it is not at all unpleasant for the person being tested, since the tube that is swallowed is the thickness of spaghetti and quite flexible.

What Are the Different Types of Motor Disturbances that Cause Problems in Swallowing?

It is convenient to divide these muscular disorders into two main groups. One we call *primary esophageal disorders*. These appear to be directly attributable to disorders arising in the esophagus. They include *achalasia,* also known as *cardiospasm,* and the important group of disorders called collectively *diffuse esophageal spasm* (or DES).

The second group are those disorders that stem from general systemic diseases in the patient. The most important ones are (1) *collagen-vascular disorders,* of which the best known is *scleroderma* (now called *progressive systemic sclerosis*), with marked thickening of the skin, and (2) *diabetes.* (I discuss the unique effects of diabetes later in this Appendix.)

How Is the Primary Group of Disorders Diagnosed?

Achalasia of the esophagus—which literally means "failure to open up"—is sometimes called cardiospasm, but this spasm has nothing to do with the heart. This term refers to the increased pressure in the lower esophageal sphincter.

The individual—usually a young person—has trouble swallowing both liquids and solids. It usually gets worse with age, but might let up at other times. These people reduce their food intake and often lose weight. They also may have chest pain, especially early on in the course of this illness, as the esophagus tries to overcome the holdup at the lower esophageal sphincter.

Although we do not know the cause of achalasia, it clearly involves an incomplete relaxation of the lower esophageal sphincter, which does not open at the appropriate time. This disorder also implies a failure of the smooth muscle of the esophagus to contract, so that the contents of our swallowed diet remain in the esophagus. The trouble seems to stem from the nerve cells in the esophageal wall itself. X-rays help determine the diagnosis by revealing a "bird beak" appearance at the lower end of the esophagus, where it joins the stomach, although with time and continued obstruction, the esophagus begins to give up, loses its contractile force, and dilates. Esophageal manometry confirms the diagnosis by showing that the lower esophageal sphincter does not open appropriately on swallowing and that ineffectual, uncoordinated waves of contractions occur in the esophagus.

When the lower end of the esophagus, especially the lower esophageal sphincter area, has been studied microscopically, pathologists have found a lack or absence of certain nerve cells, the ganglion cells, which serve as relay stations for the transmission of neural impulses. For most cases of achalasia the cause of this absence of ganglion cells is unknown; however, the cause of this disorder in Brazil, where it is known as *Chagas's disease,* is an infection with a specific micro-organism of the Bartonella group.

How Is Achalasia Treated? Does Treatment Work?

The good news is that treatment of achalasia is highly successful, working in 70 to 90 percent of patients. Treatment involves the mechanical disruption, actually tearing the muscles at the lower end of the esophagus, particularly the sphincter muscles. This is accomplished by either of two methods. One dilates and stretches the sphincter muscles with an inflatable balloon which is passed through the mouth, down the esophagus, and through the sphincter; once in place, the balloon is blown up briskly. The second method entails splitting the muscles of the sphincter by an operation called *myotomy* under general anesthesia. Both methods have approximately the same success, but nowadays the balloon technique—called *pneumatic dilation*—is the method of choice, is usually done before surgery is considered, and is quite safe. Yet the risk of perforating the esophagus—even if only a 2 to 3 percent risk—makes it clear that this procedure should be performed only by those with extensive experience and a very good track record. Sometimes balloon dilatation may need to be repeated once, twice, or more if the initial attempt has failed.

The surgical method of esophageal myotomy—the splitting of

the sphincter muscles—has of course the general risks of a major abdominal operation under general anesthesia. Its special hardship is that the disruption of the sphincter may be too "good" and lead to an open gateway of free reflux in about 18 percent of cases. Thus sometimes an antireflux operation is added to the myotomy. For this reason, surgery is usually reserved for those who have failed to recover after pneumatic stretching, perhaps after two or three trials.

From the discussion so far, you can deduce that drug treatment has little to contribute to the long-term management of a patient's achalasia. Calcium channel blockers, such as nifedipine (Procardia®), given by mouth or placed under the tongue can lower the esophageal pressure, both in normal subjects and in patients with achalasia. Nitrates—for example, isosorbide dinitrate—also relax the smooth muscle of the sphincter just as effectively, but have the disadvantage of lowering blood pressure. In general, however, drug therapy alone has a small part to play in treating this disorder. It may be useful as an additional treatment, especially if muscle-splitting or stretching procedures have been only partially effective.

Diffuse Esophageal Spasm

We have talked about diffuse esophageal spasm (DES) at some length in Chapter 7, but DES deserves further consideration since its sufferers often have two specific difficulties in swallowing that need not be closely correlated in time with their chest pains. They experience problems in swallowing liquids, as well as solids, and often have trouble after taking carbonated beverages or other liquids of extreme temperature—either hot or cold. These patients' trouble in swallowing is not as severe as those with achalasia, rarely worsens with time, and they do not lose weight.

X-rays and esophagoscopy rarely help to make the diagnosis, but esophageal manometry is critical. The waves of contraction recorded by this method often reveal high prolonged levels that are not coordinated; that is, they do not succeed each other in a progressive fashion downstream and thus do not move things through the esophagus in a smooth, undisturbed fashion.

It is occasionally difficult to demonstrate these abnormalities at the time of the pressure studies, and subjects may not experience irregularities during testing. Attempts to produce symptoms in abnormal patients by using a variety of drugs have not been too helpful. Thus, while we may arrive at a clinical diagnosis, structural difficulties must be carefully ruled out before labeling the patient a sufferer of DES, lest we miss a stricture or a congenital web.

What About the Treatment of DES?

Fortunately DES is quite rare for it is a disorder difficult to treat in contrast to achalasia; however, the drugs already mentioned can be quite useful in my experience. Obviously, very cold or hot liquids must be eliminated along with carbonated beverages. Calcium channel blockers, such as the nifedipine (Procardia®) variety, can reduce the size and force of the esophageal contractions which are not moving things along. Nitrates can reduce the pain in the chest, but seem to have little influence over abnormal contractions.

Because some patients with cardiospasm (achalasia) early in the course of the disease may have DES, and because these disorders may be related to each other, physicians have tried forceful dilatation with balloons in DES patients who have not responded to conventional drugs. About one-half of these patients improve, more in terms of their swallowing problem than in terms of their chest pain. Even esophageal myotomy has been performed over long segments of the esophagus and with some success.

I should add that some nonspecific esophageal motor disturbances exist that authorities in this field cannot fit into the clear-cut categories we have been discussing. It is thus essential that structural disorders (strictures, webs, scars, and tumors) be completely eliminated by all our imaging techniques, including in some cases CAT scanning of the lower half of the esophagus.

Difficulty in Swallowing Due to Systemic Disease

Patients with trouble swallowing must be examined from the point of view of other more generalized diseases as well. One of the most troublesome in this context is the disease scleroderma, now called *progressive systemic sclerosis*. It is easy to recognize the thickened skin of the face, forehead, and hands characteristic of this disease, which is one of a group of diseases called *collagen vascular disorders*. (This disease group also includes *lupus erythematosus, rheumatoid arthritis,* and *dermatomyositis*.) All of these disorders have a curious association with *Raynaud's phenomenon*, in which sufferers complain of sensitivity to the cold in fingers and toes. (Raynaud's syndrome is discussed more fully in the next section of this Appendix.)

At times, esophageal problems appear before the skin is altered or often before the skin changes are recognized. The major problem in swallowing stems from diminished or absent contractions in the smooth muscle of the esophagus and very low pressure in the lower esophageal sphincter, which leads to reflux, esophagitis, and ultimately to stricture. So, in this instance, functional disorder leads to structural disorder, and it is often difficult to separate one from the other. Treatment is not easy, but the prokinetic agents—metoclopramide, domperidone, and Cisapride®—may improve the emptying of the esophagus. The strictures, as they form, can be stretched by dilation.

Cold Hands and Trouble Swallowing: Raynaud's Phenomenon

"Cold hands, warm heart." We all know the old cliché. But what have cold hands to do with swallowing? Why does your doctor want to know if you have ever been considered a sufferer of Raynaud's phenomenon?

First, what is this phenomenon, named after a French doctor, Maurice Raynaud, who described it in 1862? Basically, it is extreme sensitivity of the fingers and hands, and occasionally the toes, to cold. Suddenly, on exposure to low temperatures, putting one's hand into cold water, holding an ice cube, or even after emotional stress, the sufferer, usually a relatively young woman, will notice that her hands have become ice cold, her fingers white, and numbness sets in. Next, the extremities, both right and left hands, become bluish. When attacks are over, the hands become red. All these changes are due to spasm in the blood vessels, especially the small ones of the hand, which cut down the flow of red arterial blood that carries the oxygen and gives our hands their pinkish color.

This behavior of the blood vessels, not often associated with any disease, is called *primary Raynaud's phenomenon*. While much remains to be learned about the condition, which seems to affect 2 to 5 percent of the population, there are now more devices and some medications, as well as dietary measures, which are most helpful.

The characteristic of Raynaud's phenomenon with which we are interested in this context is associated with underlying disease; in this case, it it called *secondary Raynaud's phenomenon*. We include it here because it may be a clue to trouble in swallowing. As we have already discussed, difficulty in swallowing involves a problem of motility, in the transport of material from the mouth to the stomach. This neuromuscular disturbance may occur in connection with a group of diseases called the *collagen vascular diseases*—the most common being *progressive systemic sclerosis, lupus,* and *rheumatoid arthritis*. Sometimes, this group of diseases are lumped together and labeled *mixed connective tissue* disorders. Whatever the label, fluids and solids no longer move effortlessly through the esophagus. Since the disorder affects both muscle and nerve fibers by way of the smallest blood vessels, the esophagus will become swollen by inflammation.

Often these collagen vascular diseases reveal themselves by characteristic changes, such as stiffness of the skin, as occurs in scleroderma, by muscle and joint changes, as in rheumatoid arthritis, or by a skin rash, as in lupus. At other times, they remain quite hidden, revealing themselves only by causing trouble in swallowing. If this clue is understood, it may lead to proper treatment of the underlying disease. Sometimes, the changes in the fingers may be the only sign that the difficulty in swallowing is part of an underlying disease which has yet to appear and reveal itself. That the esophagus is not working correctly can be documented by observing under the fluoroscope the lack of swallowing waves when the subject drinks. It may be recorded on motion picture films and demonstrated by a lack of pressure changes in the esophagus when these are measured.

These collagen vascular diseases damage not only the muscles of the esophagus, which sweep its contents before them, but also injure the muscles of the gatekeepers at the junction of the esophagus and stomach, the lower esophageal sphincter. This damage sets the stage for the reflux of the stomach contents, especially acid, into the esophagus, resulting in heartburn and "peptic esophagitis." This, in turn, may lead to scarring and narrowing of the interior, with the formation of a stricture, a fixed unyielding scar, which may need to be carefully stretched to allow food to get through the esophagus into the stomach.

For those who want to read more about this fascinating and unusual subject, the article by Dr. John Stone, "Why Some Hands Get So Cold," in the *New York Times Magazine* of March 2, 1989 (pages 62–64) is both enjoyable and informative.

A Little More on Delayed Stomach Emptying

Because the concept of disordered motility of the upper gastrointestinal tract, which results in the delay in stomach emptying with its accompanying host of symptoms of indigestion, is beginning to play such a large part in our current medical treatment, I want to devote a little more discussion to this area of *gastroparesis:* weakness of the stomach wall muscles.

The possible diagnostic causes of this condition are extensive. A brief outline of some of the possible ones will explain why the search for them can be difficult and tedious, and involve considerable testing and detective work.

First, there are the mechanical causes: pre-pyloric, pyloric, and duodenal ulcers which result in scarring of the pyloric channel, as well as a curious condition in the adult called *hypertrophic pyloric stenosis,* which resembles the congenital condition of pyloric stenosis of the newborn.

Second, peptic ulcer disease delays gastric emptying. About 60 percent of individuals with reflux severe enough to cause esophagitis have delayed emptying, and gastric ulcers reduce the pumping action of the antrum of the stomach.

Third, we have already discussed non-ulcer dyspepsia (Chapter 6) which also may include gastric emptying.

Fourth, some metabolic disorders, like hyperthyroidism (overactive thyroid) and hyperparathyroidism (overactivity of the parathyroid hormone which raises the blood calcium level), may result in gastroparesis.

Fifth, several drugs, such as anticholinergics like Pro-Banthine®, atropine and belladonna, nicotine, and the tricyclic antidepressants like Elavil®, interfere with the central nervous system's control of the stomach.

Some psychological disorders, such as anorexia nervosa, bulimia, and depression, may also interfere with normal stomach emptying.

Recent studies have shown that disturbances in the gastric electrical rhythm, either a rapid or too slow activity, can be involved in this condition and may require special measurements of the electrical activity of the stomach (electrogastrogram) for its demonstration (discussed in the section on nausea and vomiting in this Appendix).

The effects of one of the most common metabolic and endocrinological disorders of the human body, diabetes mellitus, deserves separate consideration because it can change the workings of the entire gastrointestinal tract.

The Strange Effects of Diabetes

Diabetes can lead to symptoms that manifest themselves along the entire gastrointestinal tract and that seem to be related to the effects of this widespread disease on muscular functions. Frequently, this aspect of diabetes is overlooked, although a considerable number of diabetic individuals complain of upper abdominal discomfort, nausea and vomiting, and occasionally have difficulty in swallowing. Yet the other complications of diabetes are well known and recognized.

As in diabetes itself, the cause of the disturbance is far from clear, but it is generally held that there is a disorder of nervous control of the gastrointestinal tract, similar to the disturbance of the nerves in other parts of the body that contribute to the diabetic complications elsewhere—such as numbness of the feet and soles, impotence in the male, and constipation or diarrhea.

Heartburn and difficulty in swallowing are not common, yet they can be most annoying when they do occur. These symptoms seem to arise from low pressures in the esophageal sphincter, which allow reflux and reduce the force of the esophageal muscle contractions in peristalsis, which interferes with the transportation of materials through the esophagus. Heartburn can be treated by the usual medications already mentioned in Chapter 4 on heartburn and peptic esophagitis. When diabetes slows the esophagus's motor activity, this can be treated by the prokinetic agents: metoclopramide, domperidone, and Cisapride®.

Delayed gastric emptying—gastroparesis—is probably the most important disorder in the stomach of diabetic persons, which leads to nausea, vomiting, weight loss, early satiety, and especially upper abdominal distention. In these individuals, the emptying of both solids and liquids is delayed. The point to remember in this connection is that upper gastrointestinal X-rays done with barium do not detect this delay. The Lord did not mean us to eat barium, which is heavier than water and has a high specific gravity, which means it moves by gravity unlike food. The specific gravity of food is close to one (like water) and is moved along by the peristaltic contractions of the stomach muscles, which develop the required increase of pressure in the stomach. It is this pressure that forces the pulverized food of the stomach to exit through the pylorus.

To detect any real delay in gastric emptying, one must rely on scanning techniques using labeled meals (solid and liquid). The details are discussed in Chapter 3 on imaging techniques. It is here that the prokinetic drugs already mentioned have their greatest usefulness. Metoclopramide is limited because of the neurological side effects it sometimes produces when it crosses the blood-brain barrier. These side effects can be avoided by the use of domperidone (Motilium®), which does not cross the blood-brain barrier. The newest of the trio, Cisapride®, has shown promise, although it has not been released by the FDA for general use. It has, however, become available in Canada and Western Europe. Interestingly enough, the antibiotic *erythromycin* has been demonstrated by Belgian workers to stimulate and improve gastric emptying in diabetic patients, especially when given intravenously; this antibiotic also seems to be somewhat effective when taken by mouth. Erythromycin deceives the receptors on the muscles of the stomach by mimicking the hormone motilin, which normally stimulates the stomach to contract.

A Controversial Aside: The Yeast Connection

Many people have chronic complaints for which modern medicine has no answers and which lead them from doctor to doctor. The trendy label of *chronic fatigue syndrome* is well known and increasing in popularity; some recent reports of viral studies of this condition may shed new light on this disabling condition.

Even better known and widely written about is the *yeast connection* which has tried to connect the presence of the fungal organism *Candida albicans,* a normal inhabitant of the human intestinal tract, with some medical problems. The most emphasized combination of symptoms, and yet still very poorly defined, is the *Candidiasis hypersensitivity syndrome*. These sufferers, according to their vocal proponents, are women with an overgrowth of *Candida albicans* on mucous membranes and intestinal linings which leads to a general toxic reaction. The women suspected of this condition have persistent vaginal infections with the organism and other gynecological symptoms.

My interest in talking about it in this book comes from the proposed idea that these syndromes can lead to many gastrointestinal symptoms which have been labeled in the past as indigestion or dyspepsia. They include abdominal bloating, nausea, indigestion, diarrhea, and abdominal pain and cramping. As a result, many women, even without vaginal candidiasis, and now men with diarrhea and other functional gastrointestinal symptoms, are treated for the presence of this organism because of indigestion or symptoms of irritable bowel syndrome; most do not carry any *Candida* in either their vaginas or their intestinal tracts.

These sufferers are usually given an antifungal medicine, Nystatin®, and advised to avoid foods containing yeast or molds and to reduce their intake of dietary sugars. There is also the claim that depression and chronic fatigue are due to the fungal syndrome.

My own feeling is that there is very little to this theory. More important, there has been very little evidence brought forth, by its supporters, of any scientific worth. The organism is present in the normal individual's gastrointestinal tract. In my experience, whether it is there or not has nothing to do with these individuals' other complaints or lack of complaints.

There is no question, however, that, in some serious conditions in which the immune system is depressed, compromised, or not functioning, these normal fungal intestinal inhabitants can enter the bloodstream, cause the condition of thrush in the mouth, and damage the kidneys. These are patients with some forms of cancer and immunological disorders, those receiving large doses of drugs which depress the immune system (such as cortisone), those on hyperalimentation who are being fed completely by vein (TPN), and especially those with the HIV virus. This is not the case in the individuals labeled as having the yeast connection.

Up to quite recently, no serious studies have been carried out in an effort to document the nature of the disease or even if it exists, especially to study in a scientific fashion the success of the proposed treatment. It may be that I see only those men and women who have failed to respond to treatment of this disorder. These are many; and I have seen some serious disorders overlooked because of this approach. Most recently, even while I was writing this very passage, a very carefully designed study of the effects of Nystatin® in women presumed to have the Candidiasis hypersensitivity syndrome showed that Nystatin®, however it was given, was no better than a placebo (a dummy pill) in improving their general symptoms or indigestion. This study will probably not end the controversy or satisfy those who support it since no dietary advice was given to test subjects.

Until further careful studies are carried out, and they certainly should be, I believe that the case for the yeast connection is not proven. I see no convincing evidence of its value for my patients.

Index